Praise for Beyond the Blues

It is a great pleasure to recommend Shoshana and Pec's "Beyond the Blues." They have designed an easy-to-use format for all practitioners who work with childbearing women. While the topic is extremely complex, their book provides the most essential information in a concise manner. This is a long overdue contribution to the field of maternal mental health. Thank you Shoshana and Pec!

— JANE HONIKMAN, MS
   FOUNDING DIRECTOR, POSTPARTUM SUPPORT INTERNATIONAL

Succinct yet informative, a useful guide for the busy practitioner or overwhelmed mother.

— VALERIE RASKIN, MD
   PSYCHIATRIST, AUTHOR OF THIS ISN'T WHAT I EXPECTED, AND
   WHEN WORDS ARE NOT ENOUGH

After reading "Beyond the Blues," I immediately ordered several copies and shared them with colleagues. It is a wonderful resource, easy to read and full of practical wisdom. I've worked with postpartum families for many years and learned a great deal reading this book.

— MAGGIE MUIR, LMFT, IBCLC
   NURSING MOTHERS COUNSEL

A comprehensive and concise guide that will enrich your understanding of perinatal mood disorders. In an easy-to-read format, Shoshana Bennett and Pec Indman have identified the essentials of risk assessment, diagnosis and treatment. A "must have" for every health practitioner who works with women at this critical time in their lives, and a necessity for every woman and family who is suffering.

— DIANA LYNN BARNES, PSY.D., MFT
PRESIDENT, POSTPARTUM SUPPORT INTERNATIONAL

As a psychotherapist treating postpartum women, I have referred to the information in this book over and over. Drs. Indman and Bennett are two reliable sources who have checked all their facts while intelligently turning this very complex topic into something so clear and understandable.

Most useful to me are the treatment protocols at the back of the book. A look of relief washes over a pregnant client's face when, together we have identified her risk factors, and chosen a course of treatment that follows these detailed protocols. For a woman who finds it difficult to be vulnerable, and accept help or care, there is something very reassuring and validating in knowing that her treatment plan is "prescribed" just for her, and will give her the best chance of preventing or working through her depression and/or anxiety. Thank you Drs. Indman and Bennett for your important contribution!

— KIM RICHARDSON, MA, LCPC
PRIVATE PRACTICE

Seminars
Training
Workshops
Consultation

Drs. Bennett and Indman offer consultation, lecture and training on perinatal illness to a wide variety of professionals and organizations. Sample topics include:

- *Assessment, diagnosis and prevention*
- *Psychotherapy models and techniques*
- *The latest research in psychopharmacology*
- *Consequences of untreated illness*
- *Resources to help suffering families*

They tailor their presentations to fit the particular needs and interests of the participants. Working individually or as a team, they can provide any type of program at your facility, from a brief lunch hour talk to a comprehensive two-day seminar. Please contact them directly for scheduling and fee information.

Their "Perinatal Mood Disorders" workshops are offered twice a year in the San Francisco Bay Area. Nurses, doctors, psychologists, marriage and family therapists and social workers can earn fourteen hours of continuing education units.

Watch for workshop and training dates on:
www.beyondtheblues.com

or contact Shoshana Bennett or Pec Indman directly:

SHOSHANA BENNETT, PH.D.	PEC INDMAN ED.D., MFT
drshosh@beyondtheblues.com	pec@beyondtheblues.com
(510) 889-6017	(408) 252-5552

I didn't know what to do when my wife started crying all the time after we came home from the hospital. The obstetrician handed me this book and finally things started making sense. It wasn't easy, but we made it through. The chapter for husbands was really useful for me because it told me what I should and shouldn't do to help my wife.

— JEFF B.
HUSBAND OF RECOVERED WIFE

This valuable treatment manual should be in the pocket of every practitioner who works with women. It is well researched and indexed for quick and easy reference by healthcare providers as well as clients and their families. As a registered nurse and lactation consultant, I have found it invaluable in assisting new mothers to comfortably achieve the breastfeeding experience they want with their babies. Thanks for dispelling so many of the old myths!

— PAT ROSS, RN, IBCLC
KAISER PERMANENTE

Before I read this book I thought I was the only mother who felt this way. It was reassuring to know that I wasn't alone! My husband read the chapter for partners and he finally knew what to say to help me. It was a relief for both of us. I'm really glad this book was written when I needed it, and I feel so sorry for all those women before me who didn't get this help.

— PATTY B.
RECOVERING MOTHER

"Beyond the Blues" is a concise, straightforward book on prenatal and postpartum depression. It addresses the questions women are reluctant to discuss with their doctors, spouses, and friends. This book is an invaluable guide not only for women experiencing these disorders, but should also be mandatory reading for all who work with women during pregnancy and postpartum. It is a true breakthrough on the topic of prenatal and postpartum depression. This is the one book you should have on your shelf.

— LISA NAKAMURA
POSTPARTUM DOULA, NURTURING MOTHER POSTPARTUM SERVICES

I never knew you could be depressed when you're pregnant. I was told that the pregnancy hormones would keep the depression away. I was severely depressed two months ago and my mother found "Beyond the Blues" for me. Now I am eight months pregnant, and I can't wait for my baby!

— CAROLE B.
EXPECTANT MOM

"Beyond the Blues" by Shoshana Bennett and Pec Indman is a very insightful, concise, informative manual that should be in the hands of all providers and new mothers dealing with postpartum depression. It is a fantastic book containing all the necessary questions and answers.

— SHIRLEY HALVORSON
PRESIDENT, DEPRESSION AFTER DELIVERY (NORTH CAROLINA)
COORDINATOR, POSTPARTUM SUPPORT INTERNATIONAL (NORTH CAROLINA)

"Beyond the Blues" is a must read for any family suffering from postpartum depression. The book provides practical, easy-to-follow advice for moms, dads, grandparents, and more. Most importantly, Shoshana and Pec paint a clear picture of this horrible illness. They provided me with a constant reminder that my wife was not alone in her suffering and would absolutely recover with proper care. The book provided hope at a time when it was hard to find.

— Mark S.
Husband of recovering wife

An extremely valuable resource guide for practitioners, as well as women and their families who are concerned about postpartum depression. Presented in an engaging and informative easy-to-understand format that both enlightens and reassures the reader. Highly recommended!

— Sarah F. McMoyler, RN, BSN, FACCE
Founder/Director, Sarah McMoyler's Birth University

I recommend this useful book to women who participate in my program and to their families, as well as to all my colleagues. It's an excellent source of information on perinatal depression in a straightforward and concise format.

— Leslie Lowell-Stoutenberg, RNC, MS
Director, Pregnancy & Postpartum Mood & Anxiety Disorder Program

About the Authors

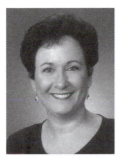

SHOSHANA S. BENNETT, PH.D. the mother of Elana and Aaron, founded Postpartum Assistance for Mothers in 1987 after her second experience with undiagnosed postpartum illness. Dr. Bennett is the president of California's state organization Postpartum Health Alliance and a coordinator for Postpartum Support International. She is a noted guest lecturer, and her work has been the subject of numerous newspaper articles around the country. Dr. Bennett has been a featured guest on national radio and television shows, including ABC's "20/20". She is a national talk radio show host on Voice America www.voiceamerica.com where her presentations are devoted mainly to perinatal topics. For fifteen years prior to her current profession, Dr. Bennett was a college instructor in the fields of Special Education, Early Childhood Development, Rehabilitation Therapies and Psychology. In addition to three teaching credentials, she holds her second masters degree in Psychology and a doctorate in Clinical Counseling. Her offices are located in the San Francisco Bay Area, and she offers telephone sessions to families throughout the country.

PEC INDMAN, ED.D., MFT has a doctorate in counseling, a masters degree in health psychology, and is licensed as a marriage and family therapist. Her training as a physician assistant in family practice was at Johns Hopkins University. Dr. Indman is secretary of Postpartum Health Alliance and a trainer for Postpartum Support International. She is a member of Depression After Delivery, the North American 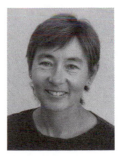 Society for Psychosocial OB/GYN and the Marcé Society, and participates in annual conferences. Dr. Indman is an editorial advisor for OBGYN.net, and has been interviewed on national radio and for several newspaper and magazine articles. Lecturing for a wide variety of audiences, Dr. Indman also provides trainings at hospitals and for organizations. She is in private practice in Santa Clara, California and is the mother of two girls, Megan and Emily.

Beyond the Blues

A Guide to
Understanding and Treating
Prenatal and Postpartum Depression

Shoshana S. Bennett, Ph.D.

Pec Indman, Ed.D., MFT

Moodswings Press

Bennett, Shoshana S.
   Beyond the blues : a guide to understanding and
treating prenatal and postpartum depression / Shoshana
S. Bennett, Pec Indman. -- 1st ed.
   p. cm.
   Includes bibliographical references and index.
   ISBN 0-9717124-1-7

   1. Postpartum depression. 2. Depression in women.
3. Pregnancy--Psychological aspects.   I. Indman, Pec.
II. Title.

RG852.B46 2003   618.7'6
                            QBI02-200725

Published in the United States
Moodswings Press, 1050 Windsor Street, San Jose, CA 95129-2837
www.beyondtheblues.com

This book is dedicated to:

Henry
by Shoshana

He suffered with me through two postpartum depressions. He brought snacks to the children upstairs, so I could lead groups downstairs. He supported my career change, and parented Elana and Aaron as I helped that career grow. He typed my doctoral dissertation, cooks and cleans more often than I do, hangs up my clothes in the bedroom, and is a really nice guy.

Ken
by Pec

With my love and appreciation for your support and encouragement of my passions. When I've flown off to attend conferences or teach, work evenings, or had meetings on the weekends, you've held down the home front. You are my partner in work, home, and play.

Contents

Foreword

How appropriate it is that I am writing this foreword as I return from the 2002 meeting of the Marcé Society in Sydney, Australia. The meeting was fascinating though intense, and covered the newest research on psychiatric illness in mothers. There is cause for great hope for childbearing women!

Beyond the Blues made excellent reading for the flight back. This fine publication fills the education void between sufferers of postpartum disorders (women, men and families) and healthcare professionals. Concise information is provided for all! Those of us who do clinical work and research in perinatal psychiatry define therapies, evaluate effects of medication for breastfeeding babies, explore preventive treatment, and much more — all very important endeavors. But the community of parents must be connected to well-informed professionals in order for even the most exciting of data to be put to use.

A very warm thank you to these two dedicated women for their commitment and sensitivity, and to Shoshana and Henry for their willingness to share the pain of their postpartum experience. It is my sincere hope that the countless people who read this book will benefit from your pain, thereby lessening the intensity of its memory.

Katherine L. Wisner, MD, MS
Professor of Psychiatry, Obstetrics and Gynecology and Pediatrics
Director, Women's Behavioral HealthCARE
Western Psychiatric Institute and Clinic/University of Pittsburgh Medical Center
University of Pittsburgh School of Medicine

Preface

Postpartum depression (PPD), the most common perinatal mood disorder, is an illness that besets a significant number of women around the world. In the United States alone, over 3.5 million women give birth each year. Since the rate of PPD is between 15 and 20 percent, about 700,000 of these women will experience postpartum depression. The rate of gestational diabetes is between 1 and 3 percent and the rate of a Downs syndrome baby occurring in a 35-year-old mother is 3 percent. Curiously, we screen routinely for these conditions, which occur less often than postpartum depression, but we do not screen for postpartum depression, which afflicts up to one in five mothers.

While working in our communities, we have been asked numerous times to provide simple guidelines for assessment and treatment of perinatal mood disorders. Mothers and their partners have been asking the question, "Why is this happening to us and what can we do about it?" Many good books and journal articles have already been written on this topic. Our main goal is to summarize this information into a practical, easy-to-use format.

This book is not meant to be used as a replacement for individual counseling, group support, or medical assessment, nor do we intend it to be a comprehensive textbook. While this book will provide critical information for psychotherapists and clients alike, it is not specifically intended to teach psycho-therapy techniques for working with perinatal clients. We want, instead, to provide the most essential and up-to-date diagnostic and treatment information as concisely as possible.

Acknowledgements

We thank Jill Wilk, a postpartum depression survivor, who generously donated her time to this effort as a labor of love. We also wish to thank Nely Coyukiat-Fu, MD, and Jules Tanenbaum, MD, for their review of the medical protocols, plus Betsy Miller and Maxine Granadino for providing our editing. To our husbands, Henry and Ken, thank you for your technical support. To our children, Elana, Aaron, Megan and Emily, for teaching us about being moms. And to our dear clients, who trust us with their deepest fears and greatest hopes.

Shoshana S. Bennett, Ph.D.
510-889-6017
drshosh@beyondtheblues.com

Pec Indman, Ed.D., MFT
408-252-5552
pec@beyondtheblues.com

Introduction

I lost my wife, Kristin Brooks Rossell, to suicide following a four-month battle with postpartum psychosis. All the things one should not do in the treatment of this deadly disease were done to Kristin. *Beyond the Blues* is a step-by-step guide that would have saved her life.

The irony is that one of the authors, Dr. Bennett, lived less than ten miles from where Kristin worked and suffered daily. Kristin was even employed at a managed healthcare company with, supposedly, decent medical insurance. But not one of the professionals in charge of her care gave her the advice and counsel needed. This book should be required reading for every expectant mother, partner, and medical person charged with the woman's care.

Beyond the Blues is not long, yet its content is comprehensive and well written. I cried reading each page, knowing at each turn how this information could have been used to save Kristin, myself, and our families the pain and needless suffering we experienced.

The single greatest gift we have is the gift of life and creation of that life. It is an indictment of our patriarchal society that a disease which afflicts over 700,000 women each year in the US alone, is not routinely screened for. "Suicide is the most preventable form of death in the US today," stated former US Surgeon General David Satcher. If this is so, and I believe it is, then surely suicide as a result of poorly treated or untreated postpartum illness is the most preventable form of suicide.

I am still in therapy and have had support from family and friends in order to deal with the loss. By founding the Kristin Brooks Hope Center I have tried to make something good come out of my personal tragedy. The Hopeline Network 1-800-

SUICIDE (784-2433) automatically connects callers — people who are depressed or suicidal, or those concerned about someone they love — to a certified crisis center. Crisis center calls are answered by trained crisis line workers 24 hours a day, seven days a week.

> *Never doubt that a small group of thoughtful,*
> *committed citizens can change the world; indeed,*
> *it's the only thing that ever has.*

MARGARET MEAD

H. Reese Butler II
CEO & Founder, Kristin Brooks Hope Center
National Hopeline Network 1-800-SUICIDE
609 E. Main St. #112
Purcellville, VA 20132

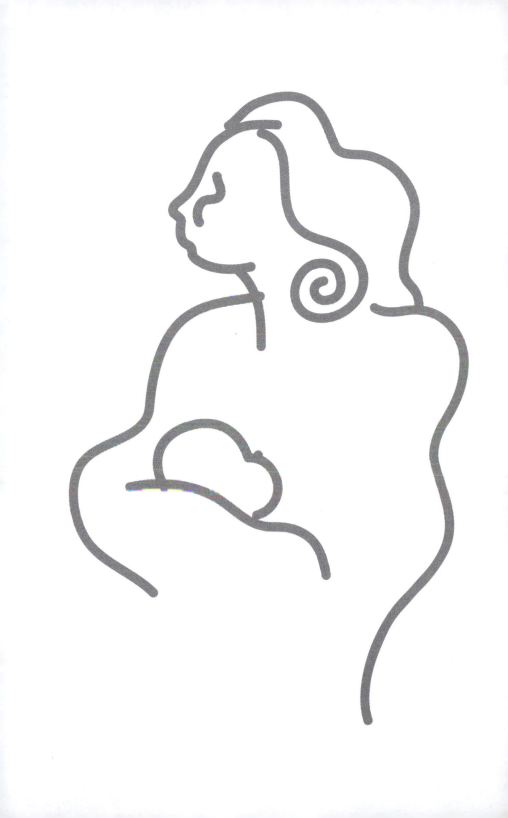

ONE

Our Stories

We arrived at this professional focus by very different paths, one through personal suffering, the other through social activism.

Shoshana's Story

My husband Henry and I happily awaited the birth of our first child. We enjoyed a wonderful marriage and had planned carefully for the addition of children to our home. We had both grown up in healthy, stable families with solid value systems. We were well-educated people with successful careers: my husband, a human resources professional, and I, a special education teacher. I had worked with children for years, beginning with my first baby-sitting job at age ten.

I felt quite confident taking care of children. The picture I had of my future always included children of my own. I prided myself on being a self-reliant person, able to manage well even under difficult circumstances. Henry came from a family of five children and had always planned on having a large family. We had many well thought-out plans for the future, and we looked forward with eager anticipation to being parents.

I felt terrific during pregnancy, both physically and emotionally. After childbirth classes, Henry and I felt prepared for the big event. There was one quick mention of C-sections and no mention at all about possible mood difficulties during pregnancy or after delivery. These classes were all about breathing techniques and what to pack in your hospital bag. On the top of every sheet on the note pad our teacher gave us appeared the words, "No drugs please." And it was also assumed, of course, that every woman would choose to breastfeed.

I endured five and a half days of prodromal labor (real labor, but unproductive), during which I could not sleep due to the discomfort. This was followed by another day of hard labor (still prodromal). My baby was transverse (sideways) and posterior ("sunny side up"), a position that caused severe back labor as well. I writhed as the sledgehammer-like pain hit to the front, then with no break, hit to the back. After not sleeping for almost a week, my insides were so sore and exhausted I thought I would literally die. At that moment a very strange thing happened. I suddenly became aware that I was hovering over myself, watching myself in pain. Although at the time I had no words to label that bizarre sensation, I now know it to be called an out-of body experience. Still not dilating, I was finally given a C-section.

My illusion of being in control was shattered. I had been a professional dancer, and my body had always done what I had wanted it to. The visual image I repeatedly had during this ghastly time was of a beautiful, perfect, clear glass ball violently exploding into millions of pieces. That was the self I felt I was losing. Hopelessness and helplessness replaced my previous feelings of control and independence. I was left with a posttraumatic stress disorder that haunted me for years.

I soon learned a skill that I would practice for a very long time — acting. I bought into the myths that I was supposed to feel instant joy and fulfillment in my role as a mother, as well as an instantaneous emotional attachment to my baby. As my daughter, Elana, was placed in my arms, I managed to say all my lines correctly. "Hi, honey, I'm so happy you're finally here," I said, wanting to feel it (as I did later on). Inside, I was numb.

Overwhelming feelings, fear, and doom intensified as my first OB appointment approached. While I drove to the doctor's office, my anxiety level rose to unimaginable heights. I pulled my car over to the shoulder of the freeway. Crouched over the steering wheel, I experienced my first panic attack. When I returned home and called to apologize for missing my appointment, I perceived only a tone of annoyance.

I had lost all the baby weight in the hospital, but just four months postpartum, I was forty pounds overweight. I had always enjoyed a wonderful working relationship with my OB, and felt that he respected me as an intelligent patient. Now, coming to his office as a hand-wringing, depressed mess, I felt embarrassed and vulnerable. As I sat in the waiting room surrounded by mothers-to-be and women cuddling their newborns, my feelings of guilt intensified. I became totally convinced that I should never have become a mother.

Though my OB was well-meaning, his technician-like manner was anything but reassuring. He focused primarily on my incision, not my huge weight gain or uncontrolled weepiness. With tremendous shame, I confessed some of my feelings to him, including, "If life's going to be like this, I don't want to be here anymore." I was shocked and hurt when he leaned back in his chair, laughed, and said, "This is normal. All moms feel these blues." He gave me his home number so I could call his wife, but he provided no referral. As my ten-minute appointment came to a close, I began to experience my first serious suicidal thoughts.

I did call his wife, who was convinced my problem was that the baby was manipulating me. I just needed to put her on a schedule. I also reluctantly joined a new-mom's group; since everyone was suggesting it, I decided to try. That was one of the most destructive actions I took. As I entered the room full of mothers cradling their babies with delight, I felt more alienated than ever.

Discussing "problems" in this group meant pondering the best way to remove formula stains from fabrics, spit-up management, and calming a fussy baby. When I mentioned that I was having a bad time, an uncomfortable silence fell. I learned later that my name had been removed from the group's baby-sitting co-op. Upon leaving the first and only group session I attended, I felt more inadequate and scared than ever. Now I knew I was the worst mother that ever walked the planet.

Another complication was breastfeeding. Although my daugh ter latched on easily, I was overcome with pain due to inflammation and bleeding. I had been one of the "good" students who had prepared her nipples before birth, just as the nurses had suggested — rubbing them with a wash cloth to toughen them up. I asked a leader from a prominent lactation organization to help me.

While the representative proved to be very helpful with suggestions about relieving the pains of breastfeeding, her emotional support immediately ended when I divulged that I would be going back to work in six months and would have to discontinue breastfeeding. She abruptly left my home. At this point I made the decision to stop breastfeeding completely, feeling like a total failure.

Life at home was frightening and unbearable. I had full-blown postpartum obsessive-compulsive disorder. Terrifying thoughts of harming my baby plagued me. I could imagine every household item possibly hurting my innocent child. Accidently tossing my baby over the second floor railing, dropping her into the fireplace, or putting her in the microwave were common worries. I would not trust myself to be alone with her. Not even my husband knew about these horrible thoughts — I could barely admit them to myself.

If I could sleep at all, I awoke in the morning in a full panic attack, wondering if I could survive another day. The simple act of watching television could turn an already dreary day into a deeper depression. The commercials portraying mothers in wavy white dresses, with naked babies in arms, taking delight in changing diapers and smiling angelically at their bundles of joy, sent me further into the depths. These were subtle reminders of the differences between all other mothers and me.

When my husband left for work, I would beg, "Don't leave me, I can't do this by myself!" He would return from work to find me in the same emotional state as when he left. I still remember my husband peering in the front window each night with that worried look, trying to see how many of us were crying. If it was just one, it was me.

Henry was frustrated with me. His mother, who had been a postpartum nurse for twenty years and who had popped out five babies of her own without the least dose of the "blues," was feeding Henry unhelpful information like, "Shoshana is a mother now. She needs to stop complaining and just do it." My respite came each evening as I tossed Henry the baby, proceeded to the driveway, jumped into the car, and sat and cried for a half-hour. There was no laughter, no humor, no friends, and no plans. There was only despair.

My mother had come to stay with us for the first three weeks. She was wonderfully supportive but even with her therapist background, she did not recognize the signs of this serious illness. For the next year I continued on my downward spiral. I allowed no emotional or physical connection with my husband. I continued to be deprived of sleep due to insomnia and anxiety, ate without experiencing much taste, and just went through the motions with my daughter. I felt buried alive with no chance of clawing my way to the surface. I began seeing a psychologist, who never once requested any historical data on depression or anxiety in my family. All she did was probe for issues in my past, and if she couldn't find a real one, she would make one up. First she blamed my grandmother, then my sister. Finally she tried to convince me that having a Cesarean delivery caused my condition. I ended up feeling "crazier" than I did when I began. I swore I would never again open up to another professional.

When Elana was two and a half years old, my anxiety and depression began to lift significantly. "Maybe I can be a mother," I heard myself saying. My hair began to curl again for the first time since the birth. I began to enjoy my food and started seeing in color again, rather than shades of gray.

As with my first pregnancy, my second was flawless and without complication. I was enjoying my daughter by then, and the thought of a second child was a delight. After two days of prodromal labor, I decided on a C-section. The newfound enjoyment and relief from depression came to a crashing halt immediately after the birth of our son, Aaron. Although I could physically take care of him, my former "I'm incompetent" feelings returned. I would easily lose my temper at Elana, who was only three and a half years old. Having been a teacher and knowing child development, I could not find words for my shame and guilt at the way I was treating her. The brief amount of time she had her mom "all there" was suddenly ripped away from her.

In 1987, when Aaron was nearly six months old, Henry excitedly called me to look at a television documentary he was watching on postpartum depression. I was awestruck as the program described the disorder, its symptoms, causes, and possible cures. At the program's conclusion, I cried for an hour, looked at my husband, and said, "That's me!" The tremendous sensation of relief that someone had at long last described the turbulent agony I had been living felt like a weight being lifted from my whole body. Equally important, I had finally heard that postpartum depression is diagnosable and treatable and that it can go away! If this condition is so common, I thought, where are all of us?

I started reading everything I could get my hands on, from all over the world, and realized that many countries were light-years ahead of the U.S. in recognizing and treating postpartum mood disorders. In my research, I came across Jane Honikman, founder of Postpartum Support International, in Santa Barbara. Jane generously offered me valuable information so that I could begin running a self-help group in the San Francisco Bay Area.

Although I was still depressed myself, I was excited about what I had been learning and wanted to share my knowledge with other sufferers and survivors. In contrast to the new-mothers' group I had attended, my group would be a safe place for women to discuss their depression and anxiety openly, without fear of judgment. I posted two flyers, one at a local supermarket, the other at my pediatrician's office. The response was thunderous! Calls came in from all over Northern California, and some from as far away as Hawaii. Every week my living room was filled with six to fifteen women, desperate for support and guidance.

I became convinced that postpartum depression needed the same support, psychological attention, and medical tools as other mental illnesses. I made the decision to begin a new career devoted to the study and treatment of postpartum mood disorders.

For the past fifteen years, the support groups, which commenced on my living room floor, have continued and flourished. As the current president of Postpartum Health Alliance, California's state organization, I am continuing to pursue my life's work.

Pec's Story

For as long as I can remember, I have been interested in political, emotional, and sociological issues as they relate to women. In the 1970s I trained as a family practice physician's assistant and worked in community-based family health clinics for a number of years. My interests varied, and my work took me to such places as women's clinics, an industry-based employee health center, a physical and fitness evaluation center, and weight management programs.

I entered a master's program in health psychology, and for the first time felt excited about school. I decided to continue and got a doctorate in counseling, getting my marriage and family therapy (MFT) license along the way. Many of my clients were referred by physicians, and much of my work with clients, particularly women, centered on issues related to health and emotional well-being.

One day, while in a physician's waiting room before a meeting, I came across a brochure from Postpartum Support International that described postpartum depression. I scribbled down the address, thinking, "I need to learn more about this." After receiving more information about PPD, I had a very mixed emotional response. I experienced sadness, extreme anger, frustration, and outrage. In all my years of training, I had learned nothing about perinatal mood disorders. I thought back to some of the women I had probably misdiagnosed. Why aren't health practitioners taught about PPD? My anger propelled me into action.

I have two daughters, and had a miscarriage in between. My second daughter was born when I was 40, after a work-up for infertility, a laparoscopy, and thanks to Clomid. My pregnancies went fairly well but both girls, each at 8.5 pounds, were delivered by C-section. The births were positive experiences. My older daughter was able to rock her new sister in a rocking chair in the recovery room as my husband, parents, and brother celebrated. I did have the "blues," yet they passed each time as my incision healed. I was fortunate to have a close friend on maternity leave at the same time, so we were together much of the time. All in all, my pregnancies, births, and postpartum experiences were positive. This only added to my outrage about PPD. All women should have the right to an emotionally and physically healthy pregnancy and postpartum experience!

My history of political activism served me well. I joined organizations and read books, attended conferences and trainings. Jane Honikman of Postpartum Support International told me about a woman in the East Bay, Shoshana Bennett, who was doing postpartum work. I called and asked if she would meet with me to make sure I was on the right track. She agreed, and we have been working together ever since.

This work has become my passion. I have never experienced so much personal and professional meaning and reward. I hope you will join us on this mission.

TWO

Pregnancy and Postpartum Psychiatric Illness

Perinatal (during pregnancy and postpartum) mood disorders are caused primarily by hormonal changes which then affect the neurotransmitters (brain chemicals). Life stressors, such as moving, illness, poor partner support, financial problems, and social isolation are certainly also important and will negatively affect the woman's mental state. Conversely, strong emotional, social, and physical support will greatly facilitate her recovery.

Any of the five postpartum mood disorders discussed in this chapter can also occur during pregnancy. These perinatal mood disorders behave quite differently from other mood disorders because the hormones are fluctuating. A woman with a perinatal mood disorder often feels as if she's "losing it," since she can never predict how she will feel at any given moment. For instance, at 8:00 A.M., she may be gripped with anxiety, at 10:00 A.M. feel almost normal, and at 10:30 A.M. become depressed and lethargic.

Our clients who have had personal histories of depression tell us that postpartum depression feels very different (and usually much worse) than depressions at other times in their lives. One of Shoshana's postpartum clients is a survivor of breast cancer. At a support group, she eloquently explained:

When I had cancer, I thought that was the worst experience I could ever have. I was wrong — this is. With cancer, I allowed myself to ask for and receive help, and expected to be depressed. My friends and family rallied around me, bringing me meals, cleaning my house, and giving me lots of emotional support. Now, during postpartum depression, I feel guilty asking for help and ashamed of my depression. Everyone expects me to feel happy and doesn't accept that this illness is just as real as cancer.

Women who experience these symptoms need to speak up and be persistent in getting proper care. In the past, these illnesses have been trivialized and even dismissed. Research has shown how important it is to treat perinatal mood disorders for the health and well-being of the mother, baby, and entire family.

The Psychiatric Issues of Pregnancy

Contrary to popular mythology, pregnancy is not always a happy, glowing experience! Approximately 10 percent of pregnant women experience depression. Of these, about 15 percent are so severely depressed that they attempt suicide.

It can be confusing that normal pregnancy experiences such as fatigue, appetite changes, and poor sleep are similar to symptoms of mood disorders. It is easy to make a blanket dismissal of these symptoms as just part of pregnancy. However, for that 10 percent, it is essential that the proper questions are asked and intervention is given when symptoms are outside the normal realm.

When symptoms of depression or other mood disorders cause limitations in the client's ability to function on a day-to-day basis, intervention is necessary. This may include traditional (counseling and medication) or nontraditional modalities (such as Yoga or acupressure), or any combination thereof. The goal is to use whatever the individual woman needs in order to feel like herself again.

Depression during pregnancy has been associated with low birth weight (less than 2,500 grams) and preterm delivery (less than 37 weeks). Severe anxiety during pregnancy may cause harm to a growing fetus due to constriction of the placental blood vessels and higher cortisol levels.

Some women become pregnant while taking psychotropic medications for depression, anxiety, and other mood problems. Many of these medications are considered acceptable during pregnancy. A practitioner who is familiar with the current research about the safety of taking medications during pregnancy should be consulted. Often it is safer to continue a medication than risk a relapse.

The rate of relapse for a major depressive disorder (MDD) in women who discontinue their medication before conception is between 50-75 percent. The rate of relapse for MDD in those who discontinue medications at conception or in early pregnancy is 75 percent, with up to 60 percent relapsing in the first trimester. In one study, 42 percent of women who discontinued medications at conception resumed medications at some time during their pregnancy. Resources listed in the back of this manual provide helpful guidelines regarding the use of medications.

Mood Disorders

There are five postpartum mood disorders. This list details each of the principal disorders, some of their most common symptoms, and risk factors. It is important to note that symptoms and their severity can change over the course of an illness.

"Baby Blues" — Not Considered a Disorder

This is not considered a disorder since the majority of mothers experience it.

- Occurs in about 80 percent of mothers
- Usual onset within first week postpartum
- Symptoms may persist up to three weeks

Symptoms
- Mood instability
- Weepiness
- Sadness
- Anxiety
- Lack of concentration
- Feelings of dependency

Etiology
- Rapid hormonal changes
- Physical and emotional stress of birthing
- Physical discomforts

- Emotional letdown after pregnancy and birth
- Awareness and anxiety about increased responsibility
- Fatigue and sleep deprivation
- Disappointments including the birth, spousal support, nursing, and the baby

Deborah's story:

For about a week and a half after my baby was born I would cry for no reason at all. Sometimes I would feel overwhelmed, especially when I was up at night with my son. Once I even thought that I had made a big mistake having a child. I felt resentment toward my husband since his life stayed pretty much the same and mine was turned upside down. When I started going to the mother's club at two weeks, I felt so relieved that all these other moms felt the same way.

Deborah's treatment:

Since Deborah was experiencing normal postpartum adjustment, she did not require any formal treatment. Her hormones were balancing out by themselves. All she needed in order to enjoy her new life was a combination of socializing with other moms, taking time to care for herself, and working out a plan of sharing child and household responsibilities with her husband.

Depression and/or Anxiety

- Occurs in 15 to 20 percent of mothers
- Onset is usually gradual, but it can be rapid and begin any time in the first year

Symptoms

- Excessive worry or anxiety
- Irritability or short temper
- Feeling overwhelmed, difficulty making decisions
- Sad mood, feelings of guilt, phobias
- Hopelessness
- Sleep problems (often the woman cannot sleep or sleeps too much), fatigue
- Physical symptoms or complaints without apparent physical cause
- Discomfort around the baby or a lack of feeling toward the baby
- Loss of focus and concentration (may miss appointments, for example)
- Loss of interest or pleasure, decreased libido
- Changes in appetite; significant weight loss or gain

Risk factors

- 50 to 80 percent risk if previous postpartum depression
- Depression or anxiety during pregnancy
- Personal or family history of depression/anxiety
- Abrupt weaning
- Social isolation or poor support
- History of premenstrual syndrome (PMS) or premenstrual dysphoric disorder (PMDD)
- Mood changes while taking birth control pill or fertility medication, such as Clomid
- Thyroid dysfunction

Lori's story:

I was so excited about having our baby girl. My pregnancy had gone smoothly. I had been warned about the "Blues," but I just couldn't shake the tears and sadness that seemed to get deeper and darker every day. My appetite was non-existent, although I forced myself to eat because I was nursing. I lost about 30 pounds the first month. At night I was having trouble sleeping. My husband and baby would be asleep but I would have one worry after another going through my head. I was exhausted. I felt like my brain had been kidnapped. I couldn't make decisions, couldn't focus, and didn't want to be left alone with the baby.

I wanted to run away. I withdrew from friends and felt guilty about not returning phone calls. I couldn't understand why I felt so bad; I had the greatest, most supportive husband, a house I loved, and the beautiful baby I had always wanted. At times I felt close to her, but at other times I felt like I was just going through the motions — she could have been someone else's child. I thought I was the worst mother and wife on the face of the earth.

Lori's treatment:

Lori began psychotherapy and also saw a psychiatrist for medication. She was started on an antidepressant and the dosage was gradually increased. Initially she took medication to help her sleep as well. She began taking regular breaks to take care of herself. She also started attending a postpartum depression support group and met other moms with similar stories. After several months she felt like herself.

Obsessive-Compulsive Disorder

- 3 to 5 percent of new mothers develop obsessive symptoms

Symptoms
- Intrusive, repetitive, and persistent thoughts or mental pictures
- Thoughts often are about hurting or killing the baby
- Tremendous sense of horror and disgust about these thoughts (ego-alien)
- Thoughts may be accompanied by behaviors to reduce the anxiety (for example, hiding knives)
- Counting, checking, cleaning or other repetitive behaviors

Risk factors
- Personal or family history of obsessive-compulsive disorder

Tanya's story:

Each time I went near the balcony I would clutch my baby tightly until I was in a room with the door closed. Only then did I know he was safe one more time from me dropping him over. The bloody scenes I would envision horrified me. Passing the steak knives in the kitchen triggered images of my stabbing the baby, so I asked my husband to hide the knives. I never bathed my baby alone since I was afraid I might drown him.

Although I didn't think I would ever really hurt by baby son, I never trusted myself alone with him. I was terrified I would "snap" and actually carry out one of these scary thoughts. If my baby got sick it would be all my fault, so I would clean and clean to make sure there were no germs. Although I had always been more careful than other people, now I would check the locks on the windows and doors many times a day.

Tanya's treatment:

After meeting with Tanya twice individually, her therapist suggested that her husband join her in the next session. Tanya needed reassurance that her husband knew she wasn't "crazy" and would never really harm the baby. She did not want to tell him the specific graphic thoughts, so she referred to them generally as "scary thoughts." After being educated, her husband's aggravation with her being "nervous all the time" subsided.

Tanya started taking an antidepressant and within two weeks the scary thoughts were occurring far less frequently. Her therapist suggested that she wait another few weeks to join a support group since she was still too vulnerable to hear about the anxieties of others. In the meantime, she was given the names and numbers of a few women to connect with who had survived this disorder.

Panic Disorder

- Occurs in about 10 percent of postpartum women

Symptoms

- Episodes of extreme anxiety
- Shortness of breath, chest pain, sensations of choking or smothering, dizziness
- Hot or cold flashes, trembling, palpitations, numbness or tingling sensations
- Restlessness, agitation, or irritability
- During attack the woman may fear she is going crazy, dying, or losing control
- Panic attack may wake her up

- Often no identifiable trigger for panic
- Excessive worry or fears (including fear of more panic attacks)

Risk factors

- Personal or family history of anxiety or panic disorder
- Thyroid dysfunction

Chris's story:

At about three weeks postpartum I stopped leaving my house at all except for pediatrician appointments. I was afraid I might have a panic attack in the store and not be able to take care of my baby. I never knew when that wave would begin washing over me and I would "lose it." The windows had to be open all the time or else I thought I would suffocate if I had an attack.

The first time I had a panic attack I thought I was having a major heart attack. A friend drove me to the emergency room and the doctor on call told me it was only stress. He gave me some medicine but I was too afraid to take it. I went home feeling stupid, like I had made a big deal out of nothing.

Everyone told me that breastfeeding would relax me, but it did just the opposite. I never knew how much milk my baby was getting and that really worried me. Sometimes when my milk would let down I would get a panic attack. The first therapist I saw told me I must have had issues bonding with my own mother, but I knew that wasn't true and I didn't see that therapist again. On many nights I woke up in a sweat, with my heart beating so fast and hard. My head was racing with anxious thoughts about who would take care of the baby when I die. I thought I was going crazy. I was so scared.

Chris's treatment:

Chris had her first therapy appointment over the telephone since she felt she could not go outside. Her therapist talked her through taking a bit of the medication her MD prescribed, so Chris would know she had something that would help in an emergency.

Driving was too scary for her, especially in tunnels and over bridges. Her husband drove her to her next session, following a route that avoided those obstacles. Chris needed to sit near the door during the appointment just in case she felt the need to run outside for some air. Her therapist urged her to sleep for at least half the night, every night. Chris's husband began taking care of his baby for the first half of the night on a regular basis. Chris noticed immediately how sleep lowered her stress level. She attended a stress management class which also helped.

Psychosis

- Occurs in one to two per thousand
- Onset usually two to three days postpartum
- This disorder has a 5 percent suicide and 4 percent infanticide rate

Symptoms

- Visual or auditory hallucinations
- Delusional thinking (for example, about infant's death, denial of birth, or need to kill baby)
- Delirium and/or mania

Risk factors

- Personal or family history of psychosis, bipolar disorder, or schizophrenia
- Previous postpartum psychotic or bipolar episode

Mike's story:

My wife, Gloria, had a great pregnancy and a long labor. We were thrilled to have our first child, a son. But within days of his birth my wife began to withdraw into her own world. She became less and less communicative and she became more and more confused and suspicious. I almost had to carry her into the therapist's office; by that time she could hardly speak or answer questions, nor write her name on the forms her therapist gave us. I was told to take her to the hospital immediately.

When we arrived at the hospital, she became fearful and then violent. She ended up in restraints. Fortunately, she responded pretty quickly to the anti-psychotic medication, and was able to come home after about a week. She continued to improve, and when she was back to herself again, she slowly weaned off all the medications.

We had always wanted two kids, so we consulted with our therapist and psychiatrist. With careful planning, we now have our second child with a very different story to tell.

Gloria's treatment:

After being released from the hospital, Gloria continued therapy and saw the psychiatrist, who carefully monitored her medication. She worked to understand and process what had happened to her. Eventually she joined a postpartum support group which was quite helpful. Since there were no other moms present in the group who had experienced a postpartum psychosis, the group leader gave her the names and numbers of women who had "been there" and who wanted to help.

Posttraumatic Stress Disorder

• There is no available data regarding the prevalence or onset

Symptoms
• Recurrent nightmares
• Extreme anxiety
• Reliving past traumatic events (for example, sexual, physical, emotional, and childbirth)

Risk factors
• Past traumatic events

Jennifer's story:

During the delivery it all came flooding back. I felt terrorized and vulnerable. I thought I had already dealt with the abuse in my childhood. It seemed that all the years of therapy were a waste of time and money. I was so embarrassed for losing control during labor. I was angry that what happened to me as a kid was still affecting me after all this time.

My therapist told me the nightmares and flashbacks would go away but I just didn't know. It was so real — like the abuse was happening again over and over. I couldn't even leave my poor husband alone with my baby. I got the sick feeling that I couldn't even trust him. I was so messed up. I thought maybe I'd never be a normal mother.

Jennifer's treatment:

Jennifer hired a postpartum doula who took care of her and the baby for two months. Having this trusted female companion with her almost everywhere she went gave Jennifer comfort. She began weekly therapy sessions and eventually joined a support group. She and her therapist agreed that she did not need medication at this point.

Consequences of Untreated Mood Disorders

Maternal depression was placed at the top of the list entitled, "Most significant mental health issues impeding children's readiness for school" (Mental Health Policy Panel, Department of Health Services, 2002). There is a tremendous amount of data regarding the profoundly negative impact of untreated maternal depression on infants, toddlers, preschoolers, school age children and adolescents. There is an increased incidence of childhood psychiatric disturbance, behavior problems, poor social functioning, and impaired cognitive and language development. When a depressed mother goes untreated, every member of the family and all the relationships within the family are affected. The quicker the mother is treated, the better the prognosis for the entire family.

Perinatal Loss

No matter how a pregnancy is terminated, whether by nature or by choice, depression and anxiety commonly follow. Not only should grief be addressed through counseling, but medications may also be useful in reducing symptoms due to loss and hormonal changes.

When a stillbirth or neonatal death occurs, depression is, of course, to be expected. Counseling for the couple will be helpful, and medications may be needed to treat anxiety and depression. These women need to be monitored carefully for emotional symptoms in subsequent pregnancies and the postpartum period.

THREE

Women with Postpartum Disorders

In the chapters to follow, we will discuss the role of practitioners, partners, and other family members in helping mothers recover. This chapter is for you, the sufferers.

Among the women we treat are those in the healthcare and educational professions, such as MDs, nurses, daycare and preschool providers, teachers, and therapists, to name a few. We often hear from these women, "This can't be happening to me! I take care of everyone else in crisis." What we tell them is that our hormones don't care what we do for a living! No one is immune. No matter what the educational or socioeconomic level, culture, religion, or personality, wherever women are having babies, the statistics remain consistent.

Women who suffer postpartum emotional difficulty experience their anguish in many different ways. Here are some of the common feelings they express:

No one has ever felt as bad as I do.

I'm all alone. No one understands.

I'm a failure as a woman, mother, and wife.

I'll never be myself again.

I've made a terrible mistake.

I'm on an emotional roller coaster.

I'm losing it.

Please know that each woman may experience these feelings at varying levels. Some may feel all of them, and others may feel only a few. You might also recognize some of your symptoms listed in Chapter 2.

Finding a Therapist

We encourage you to contact Postpartum Support International (PSI) at (805) 967-7636 or www.postpartum.net to locate a therapist who has shown interest and commitment in the postpartum field. PSI, along with other organizations in the Resources section, provides specialized training in perinatal mood disorders. We have not found any graduate training that covers this material. Do not assume (as many insurance companies would like you to believe) that someone who has expertise in working with depression or other mood disorders is knowledgeable about perinatal mood disorders.

Sometimes an insurance company is willing to add a specialist to its provider list or pay for you to see one. If your insurance company will pay only if you see providers on their list, here are screening questions to help you determine their knowledge in this area. It's important to ask these questions, even if the therapist considers himself or herself knowledgeable. If you don't have the energy to deal with the insurance company or to screen professionals, ask a support person to do this for you.

- *What specific training have you received in postpartum mood disorders?*
- *Do you belong to any organization dedicated to education about perinatal mood disorders?*
  Someone committed to working in this field should belong to at least one of these organizations: Postpartum Support

International, Postpartum Health Alliance, Depression After Delivery, Marcé Society, North American Society for Psychosocial OB/GYN.

- *What books do you recommend to women with postpartum depression or anxiety?*
  Someone with expertise should be able to name several books listed in the Resources section of this manual.

- *What is your theoretical orientation?*
  Research has shown the most effective types of therapy for your condition are cognitive-behavioral and interpersonal. You are experiencing a life crisis; long-term intensive psychoanalysis is not appropriate.

If you are unable to find a therapist with expertise, interview until you find someone who is compassionate and willing to learn. If you do not think a practitioner is helping you, move on! Be a good consumer. Shop around until you feel satisfied that you are in capable hands.

The Truth of the Matter

As you face the challenge of a postpartum mood disorder, remind yourself of these truths:

- *I will recover!*
  We have never met a woman who, after proper treatment, did not recover.

- *I am not alone!*
  One in five women will experience a postpartum reaction more severe than the "Baby Blues."

- *This is not my fault!*
  You did not create this; it is a biochemical illness.

- *I am a good mom!*
  Even if you are hospitalized, you are still making sure your baby is provided for. The fact that you are trying to improve the quality of your life and your family's proves you are a good mom.
- *It is essential for me to take care of myself!*
  It is your job to take care of yourself so you can get better and take care of your family.
- *I am doing the best I can!*
  No matter what your current level of functioning, you are taking steps, regardless of how small they seem. Good for you!

Depression may interfere with your ability to believe these statements, so it is important to say them frequently, as if you really mean them. As you recover, this exercise will become easier.

Basic Mom Care

Finding Support People

Very often when we are in crisis, we overlook the people around us who can be of help and support. People can support you in different ways. Support may be physical; for instance, cooking, cleaning, caring for the baby, shopping, taking you for a walk or to an appointment. Emotional support may include sitting and listening, hugging, and giving encouraging words.

Even though the following writing task may feel over-whelming, it can serve to create your lifeline. This is a brain-storming exercise — write down everyone who comes to mind, regardless of the type of support they may be able to give you. If possible, do this exercise with a support person. Keep this list of supporters' names and phone numbers handy by your phone for times of need.

Here are some places where our clients have found people for their support network:

- Partner
- Family and extended family
- Neighbors
- Co-workers
- Religious communities
- Professionals (including doulas, lactation consultants, nannies, housekeepers)
- Hotlines
- Internet chat rooms (Warning: If you are anxious or obsessive we do not recommend)
- Postpartum depression support groups

Eating

Often women with postpartum depression and anxiety crave sweets and carbohydrates. If you can eat something nutritious, especially protein, each time you feed the baby, you can help keep your blood sugar level even. This will contribute to keeping your mood stable. We understand this may be difficult if you are experiencing a lack of appetite, so do the best you can. If you have trouble eating, try drinking your food — for example, protein shakes or drinks. Avoid caffeine.

Ask a support person to stock your refrigerator with things like yogurt, sliced deli meat and cheese, hardboiled eggs, pre-cut vegetables, and fruit. Better yet, if they are not already offering, ask people to bring you food. Don't forget to drink water-dehydration can increase anxiety. Appetite problems are quite common with postpartum depression and anxiety. Please tell your health practitioner about any appetite changes. It might be helpful to consult a nutritionist who is familiar with depression and anxiety when you have the energy.

Sleeping

Nighttime sleep is the most valuable sleep in helping you recover. Five hours of uninterrupted sleep per night is required for brain restoration because it gives you a full sleep cycle. The baby can be fed with breast milk or formula in a bottle. You need to be "off duty" physically, emotionally, and psychologically. You can either split the night with your partner or alternate taking a full night "on," then a full night "off."

If your partner is not home, you will need to enlist a support person to be responsible for the baby during this time. When you are "off" you should sleep away from the baby in another room, with earplugs. Many of our clients also use a fan, air purifier, or another appliance to block all baby noises. When your partner is "off," he can use the same techniques.

Remember, it is your job to take care of yourself. Even if you cannot arrange for this nightly, a few nights a week will help. If you are able to nap in the day, do so, but it does not replace nighttime sleep. Sleep problems occur frequently with mood disorders. If you are unable to sleep at night when everyone else is sleeping, please talk to your health practitioner. Medication will be helpful.

Exercising

Even a few minutes of brisk physical activity can help your mood. When you are physically able to be active, find something you are willing to do (for example, walking, dancing, or bike riding). Even if the thought of walking around the block is overwhelming, don't feel like a failure. It will get easier as you feel better. If you know you would feel better if you did the activity, but it is hard to mobilize yourself, designate a support person to encourage you and participate with you.

When you have insomnia or are very sleep-deprived, do not do intense aerobics — this can actually make your sleep condition worse. Wait until you have had at least a couple of weeks of good sleep before you resume or begin a heavy exercise program.

Taking Breaks

The myth is that if we really love our children enough, we don't need breaks from them. This certainly isn't the case! We've bought into the idea that taking time for ourselves is selfish and bad, and therefore we feel guilty when we even think we need a break. The truth is that all good mothers take breaks — that's how they stay good mothers! We strongly recommend that you get regularly scheduled time off at least three times a week for a minimum of two hours at a time. For every job other than being a mother, breaks are mandated by law, and you'd expect much more time off.

If you don't recharge your batteries, you'll be running on empty. You are not the only one who can care for the baby. Partners and family members, for instance, should be given alone time to bond with the baby too. This experience is important for the baby, and it can be done more easily with you somewhere else. Everyone wins.

If you're too depressed or tired to actually leave the house, go to another room and use earplugs or earphones. Or, maybe your support person can leave the house with the baby and give you alone time.

Going Outside

When we're depressed or anxious, the four walls feel as if they're closing in. Our world feels darker and smaller. We tend to fold in emotionally and physically (as in crossing our arms, hunching over, and fixing our gaze downward).

To counter this, go outside your home, look up at the sky, stand up straight, put your arms at your sides, and breathe. You don't have to actually go anywhere. Just go outside once a day, even if this means standing outside your front door in your bathrobe.

Taking Care of the Baby

Depending on the level of depression, you may need someone to do most, if not all, of the baby care. A support person can be with you when your partner is not, such as a family member, doula, nanny, or friend. Very gradually you can increase your participation with the baby care as your support person keeps you company.

Even though you may feel like a robot at first, just going through the motions without joy, it is still good for you to experience yourself doing "mommy" tasks. Your feelings of competence and confidence will increase, and eventually you will be able to enjoy your day.

Scripts

You may not know what you need when a support person asks, "What can I do?" It's all right to say, "I don't know what I need right now. I just know I feel awful." However, don't assume anyone can read your mind. You are most likely to get what you need if you ask for it.

Try giving your partner, family, and friends a script to guide them in how to best support you. For example, when you are experiencing anxiety, it will not be helpful to hear, "Just calm down and relax." Instead, try giving them suggestions of what to say and do:

I am sorry you are suffering.

We will get through this.

I am here for you.

Hug.

This will pass.

A script does not detract from the genuineness of caring and love. On the contrary, it will give your support people an effective way to give you what you need. People who love you want you to get better. They will be relieved to know what will help.

For Women with Anxiety or Obsessions

Be sure to avoid caffeine and keep your blood sugar level even (see section above on eating). For many women with anxiety or obsessions, information provides fuel for worry. Turn off the TV news, and don't read the news section of the newspaper. Don't read books, magazines, or Internet information about postpartum mood disorders if you find it makes you more anxious. If you go to the movies, select comedies. Find activities that can soothe or distract you, rather than those that stir up anxiety.

Stimulation

When the usual sights, sounds, and daily activity feel like too much, it is important to adjust your surroundings. Remember, you are in recovery. Treating yourself with "kid gloves" can greatly boost your recovery. Don't push yourself. If, for instance, going to a family event (even if you have had fun at this event in the past) seems overwhelming, you probably should not go. Trust yourself. As you recover, you'll be able to handle more.

When very anxious, perinatal women often feel hypersensitive to stimulation of all kinds — visual, auditory, and kinesthetic (touch). If this is happening, it may be soothing to lower the light in your house. (If you are feeling more depressed than anxious, try brightening your house with more light — open your curtains and add lamps, for example.) As long as you can hear what you need to, try wearing earplugs or earphones during the day to muffle unnecessary noise. You may become more sensitive to touch — for instance, clothing may rub, scratch or itch. Be compassionate with yourself and do what you need to in order to be comfortable.

Myths About Nursing and Bonding

Myth: *"I can't be a good mom unless I nurse my baby."*

The truth is there is no one right way to feed your baby. Whatever works for you and your family is the right way. There is a tremendous amount of pressure on new moms in our society to nurse exclusively, regardless of physical or emotional obstacles. We believe that one size never fits all. Whether you feed your baby breast milk or formula has no relationship to how much you love your child or what kind of mother you are.

There are advantages and disadvantages to both breast-feeding and bottlefeeding, and some combination of the two may work for you as well. For instance, having a support person bottlefeed with formula or breast milk so you can be off duty is a responsible choice for your family's well-being. Don't allow yourself to be guilt-tripped!

Be prepared for intrusive and inappropriate questions and comments about how you're feeding your baby. This may happen anywhere; for example, out in public, at your health practitioner's office, a mom's group, or at a family gathering. If any person, whether lay or professional, seems judgmental about the plan you've chosen, remind yourself that you have made the best decision you can for you and your family. You can ignore the question or comment or change the subject. Alternatively, you can say, "It's none of your business," "I can't breastfeed. I have a life-threatening illness," "I chose not to," or "My doctor told me I can't."

Remember, you are entitled to respond any way you need to in order to get inquisitors off your back. You have nothing to apologize about. Good moms make sure their babies are fed. Period.

Myth: *"My baby won't bond if I don't nurse."*

If this were true, there would be whole generations of adults who never bonded with their mothers! Some women actually begin to bond with their babies when they stop breastfeeding. For women who are experiencing anxiety or pain related to breastfeeding, bottlefeeding may allow this time together to be more relaxed and enjoyable. There are no rules about how to bottlefeed. If you desire skin-to-skin contact, you can bottlefeed bare-chested.

Myth: *"My baby can sense my depression or anxiety."*

Your baby cannot read your mind! Your thoughts or feelings will not damage your baby or the relationship with your baby. What babies can sense is temperature, hunger, wetness, and physical contact. Your baby will feel close to you regardless of depressed or anxious thoughts running through your head.

Myth: *"Bonding happens immediately at birth."*

No adopted children would ever bond with their adoptive moms if this were true. There is no one magic moment of opportunity when bonding must happen, and no reason to worry about bonding if you were unable to touch or hold your baby immediately after delivery. Even if your depression or anxiety has made it difficult for you to care for your baby, it's never too late. Bonding is a process of familiarity, closeness, and comfort that continues for years.

Recovery

What will help each woman recover from postpartum depression depends on the reason(s) for her illness and her preferences for treatment. Whatever helps you get better is what we recommend. In Chapter 7 we outline a few different treatment options which you may choose to do separately or in combination. Since medication is among the most common treatments for these disorders, we've listed a few of the questions we hear most often.

Antidepressant
Questions and Answers

Question: *I'm afraid medication will change my personality.*

Answer: Depression and anxiety change your personality — people who are usually easygoing and stable may become irritable, moody, withdrawn, or worried. As the medication begins to work, you will begin to feel like yourself again. In a sense, medication restores you to your "old" personality.

Question: *How long will I have to take the medicine?*

Answer: Treatment length varies, and is a decision between you and your prescribing practitioner. If this is your first episode of depression/anxiety, the general recommendation is to take a dose that gets you "back to yourself," then continue on the medicine for a minimum of six months. If you have a history of depression or anxiety, your practitioner may suggest a longer course of treatment. Staying on the medication for the recommended time is critical to reduce your chances of having a relapse or reoccurrence of illness.

Question: *Will I become dependent on the antidepressant?*

Answer: Antidepressants are not addictive or habit-forming.

Question: *What if I have side effects?*

Answer: Many people experience no side effects at all. If side effects do occur, they are usually mild and temporary, lasting less than a week (nausea, fatigue, or shakiness, for instance). If you experience a decrease in libido, it may persist through the course of treatment. If you feel more severe side effects or side effects that do not clear up after a week, contact your practitioner. Some women need to try more than one anti-depressant before they find the one that works best for them. To reduce the likelihood of side effects, it is helpful to start at a very low dose and slowly work up to the correct therapeutic dosage for you.

Question: Which antidepressant is the right one for me?

Answer: In general, most people do well on most of the medications. If you have previously been on a medication that was helpful, or if you have a blood relative doing well on a medication, that one would probably be the first choice. If you are anxious, a medication that may have a calming effect might be chosen. If you have fatigue, a medication that is energizing may be tried. The most important indicator is whether you begin to feel better.

Question: When will I feel better? How will I know if the medication is working?

Answer: Most of the newer antidepressants begin working within two weeks, while the older medications can take four to six weeks to work. Here are some comments we have heard as the medicine begins working:

I'm not crying all the time.

I have more patience — my fuse is longer.

I'm singing in the shower again.

My husband noticed I seem happier.

I feel more motivated — I'm cooking for the family again.

I'm enjoying the baby more.

I'm not worrying as much — the little things aren't getting to me.

Question: Won't medication be a crutch?

Answer: A crutch is a temporary tool that you use until you no longer need it. If you broke your foot you wouldn't think twice about using crutches to support you while your foot heals. Medication restores your brain chemistry to a normal state, allowing you to get back to feeling yourself and back to your life. As you become well you will wean off the medication.

Question: *I want to breastfeed but I don't want to take anything that will harm my baby. Can I take medication and nurse?*

Answer: According to the professionals who have dedicated their careers to studying the safety of antidepressants and nursing, the answer is yes. When infant blood was examined, few, if any, metabolites of medication were found. Babies exposed to medication through nursing are as healthy and normal in all ways as babies not exposed.

It's clear from the research that it is more important for a mom to receive proper treatment than whether she feeds her baby breast milk or formula. So if you think you will worry too much about your baby if you continue breastfeeding while taking an antidepressant, it is better to wean (slowly) rather than to go without treatment. Remember that the best gift you can give your baby is a happy, healthy mom. Often the anxiety about nursing while taking a medication goes away once the medication starts working, since the anxiety can be caused by the mood disorder itself.

Question: I am pregnant and really depressed. Do I need to feel this way for the rest of my pregnancy?

Answer: About 10% of women experience depression in pregnancy. Getting treatment is important for both you and the baby. Researchers have begun looking at the harmful effects of untreated depression and anxiety on the fetus. Also, if you are depressed or anxious in pregnancy, you may not be eating or sleeping as well as you should. This is not good for you or your developing baby.

Counseling alone may be sufficient, but often medication is necessary. SSRIs (selective serotonin reuptake inhibitors) have been shown to be helpful for both depression and anxiety. No increased risk of miscarriage or malformations has been shown to result from taking these medications, even in the first trimester. Depression in pregnancy also puts you at high risk for postpartum depression. Being on medication through pregnancy and postpartum will significantly decrease this risk.

Question: *I am embarrassed and ashamed about taking medication. Am I weak because I need a medication?*

Answer: There is a stigma in our culture about people who take psychotropic medication. This stigma is based on ignorance. Somehow it is presumed we can control our brain chemistry. If you had diabetes or a thyroid disorder you wouldn't expect (and no one would suggest) that you could will yourself to make more insulin or thyroid hormone. It's a strength to get help when we need it, not a weakness!

Taking medication is a personal choice. You are not required to share this information with others. Being private is not the same as being ashamed. However, once our clients begin to tell close family or friends, they are often surprised to find out how many of them are also on medication, or know someone who is. Whether you choose to take an antidepressant or not, find people who will support your choices for wellness.

FOUR

Partners

This chapter is designed to provide support to you, the partner, regardless of your gender or marital status. To avoid confusion, we sometimes refer to the new mother as "wife." The sooner you become involved in the recovery process, and the greater your involvement, the more you both will benefit — together and separately. The more you understand what she is experiencing, the better supported she will feel. That will, in turn, expedite her recovery.

Things to Keep in Mind

- *You didn't cause her illness and you can't take it away.*
  Postpartum depression and anxiety is a biochemical disorder. It is no one's fault. When her brain chemistry returns to normal, she will feel like herself again. It is your job to support her as this happens.
- *She doesn't expect you to "fix it."*
  Many partners feel frustrated because they feel inadequate or unable to fix the problem. She doesn't need you to try to take the problem away. This isn't like a leaky faucet that can be repaired with a new washer. Don't suggest quick-fix solutions. This isn't that kind of problem. She just needs you to listen.

- *Get the support you need so you can be there for her.*
  We frequently see the phenomenon of the partner becoming depressed during or after his wife's depression. You can avoid this by taking care of yourself and getting your own support from friends, family or professionals. You should make sure to get breaks from taking care of your family. Regular exercise or other stress-reducing activity is important, so you can remain the solid support for your wife. Provide a stand-in support person for her while you're gone.

- *Don't take it personally.*
  Irritability is common with postpartum depression/anxiety. Don't allow yourself to become a verbal punching bag. It's not good for anyone concerned. She feels guilty after saying hurtful things to you. If you feel you didn't deserve to be snapped at, explain that to her calmly.

- *Just being there with and for her is doing a great deal.*
  Being present and letting her know you support her is often all she'll need. Ask her what words she needs to hear for reassurance, and say them to her often.

- *Lower your expectations.*
  Even a non-depressed postpartum woman cannot realistically be expected to cook dinner and clean house. She may be guilt-tripping herself about not measuring up to her own expectations and worrying that you will also be disappointed. Remind her that parenting your child and taking care of your home is also your job, not just hers. Your relationship and family will emerge from this crisis stronger than ever.

- *Let her sleep at night.*
  She needs five hours of uninterrupted sleep per night to complete a full sleep cycle and restore her biorhythms. If you want your wife back quicker, be on duty for half the night without disturbing her. Many dads and partners have expressed how much closer they are to their children because of nighttime caretaking. If you can't be up with the baby during the night, hire someone who can take your place. A temporary baby nurse will be worth her weight in gold.

What to Say, What Not to Say

Say:

- *We will get through this.*
- *I'm here for you.*
- *If there is something I can do to help you, please tell me.*
  For example, care for the baby, run her a warm bath, put on soothing music.
- *I'm sorry you're suffering. That must feel awful.*
- *I love you very much.*
- *The baby loves you very much.*
- *This is temporary.*
- *You'll get yourself back.* As she recovers, point out specifics about how you see her old self returning; such as, smiling again, more patience, or going out with her friends.
- *You're doing such a good job.* Give specific examples.
- *You're a great mom.* Give specific examples, such as "I love how you smile at the baby."
- *This isn't your fault. If I were ill, you wouldn't blame me.*

Do Not Say:

- *Think about everything you have to feel happy about.*
  She already knows everything she has to feel happy about. One of the reasons she feels so guilty is that she is depressed despite these things.
- *Just relax.*
  This suggestion usually produces the opposite effect! She is already frustrated at not being able to relax despite all the coping mechanisms that have worked in the past. Anxiety produces hormones that can cause physiological reactions, such as an increased heart rate, shakiness, visual changes, shortness of breath, and muscle tension. This is not something she can just will away.

- *Snap out of it.*
  If she could, she would have already. She wouldn't wish
  this on anyone. A person cannot snap out of any illness.
- *Just think positively.*
  It would be lovely if recovery were that simple! The nature
  of this illness prevents positive thinking. Depression feels
  like wearing foggy, dark, distorted lenses which filter out
  positive input from the environment. Only negative, guilt-
  ridden interpretations of the world are perceived. This illness
  is keeping her from experiencing the lighter, humorous, and
  joyful aspects of life.

From a Dad Who's Been There

This was written by Henry, Shoshana's husband, for Shoshana's newsletter, soon after her first depression had subsided:

*You've just come home from a long day at work, hoping
to find a happy home — and what you find makes you want to
get back into the car and leave. Your wife is in tears, the baby
is crying. The house is a mess, and forget about dinner. By
now you know better than to ask how her day was. Her
response is always the same. "I hate this 'mother' stuff. I don't
want to be anyone's mother. I want my old life back. I want to
be happy again." You shrug, go to hold the baby, and wonder
why your wife is feeling this way, why she's not as happy as
you are about the baby, and when she will snap out of it.*

*You're not alone. I lived with this scene every day for two
years. Every ounce of my patience was tested, but I kept
hoping that things would be "normal" again. I focused on my
baby daughter, the one in the midst of this mess, and kept
telling myself I'd be there for her.*

*Slowly, slowly, my wife recovered from the illness. Today,
we have that happy home we both always wanted. Be patient
and tolerant. Remember, it will get better.*

FIVE

Siblings, Family, and Friends

After the birth of a baby there are many changes that occur in a household. Although older children may expect some of these changes, they probably will not be expecting Mom to be different. Even siblings who are too young to understand the concept of depression will most likely notice that their mother's behavior has not been normal.

Children usually notice if Mom is, or has been, crying. They will notice if Mom yells or gets angry over little things. Perhaps they will notice that Mom stays in bed more, does not have the energy to take them to the park, or does not seem to laugh much lately. Maybe they see her staring blankly into space, not paying much attention to them. Children can tell this is not the Mom they used to know, and they need honest, clear explanations about what is occurring.

It is crucial that the path of communication with children is open. Whenever possible the mother herself should talk with her children. The partner or another adult can help to reinforce the information. There are several important guidelines in communicating with children about what is happening.

Communicating with Children About Postpartum Depression

- Even adults are often unclear about words like "depression" or "anxiety." Instead, use descriptive words like "sad," "cranky," "tired," "weepy," "worried," or "grouchy."

- Reassure them often that they did not cause Mommy's illness or problem; this is not their fault, nor could they have done anything to prevent it.
- Let them know it is not the kind of illness caused by germs. She did not catch it from anyone, nor can she pass it on to them.
- Let the children know that Mom is getting help: seeing a doctor or counselor, taking medicine, and she will get better soon. Let them know Mom may have some good and some bad times as she recovers.
- Ask the children how they can help Mom. Perhaps they can draw a pretty picture, leave "I love you" notes around the house for her, and offer to help with age-appropriate tasks.
- Tell the truth. Children know if Mom is not "herself," so don't tell them she is fine when she is not. Mom should be direct and honest too. For instance, when it is apparent that she is feeling sad, she can say so. Sadness is just a feeling; it does not have to be logical or rational. Feelings are part of being human. To hide sadness (for example, saying, "Oh, these are 'happy tears'"), gives the message that it is not permissible to be sad.

    What we can teach our children by showing feelings is how to express ourselves in appropriate ways. This will not damage them. On the contrary, it can model behavior that will serve them well in the future. And by getting help we teach our children that when there is something wrong we can do something about it.

Here is an example of what a mother could say to her child/children:

You may have noticed I have been crying and getting mad a lot lately. Some of the chemicals in my body are not working right, and it has been affecting how I feel and how I act. I want you to know I love you very much, and I love the baby, too. I also want you to know that this is not your or anybody else's fault. I am taking good care of myself and getting help so I can get better as fast as I can. I am probably going to have good times and bad times, but I will get better and better until I'm completely well. I am looking forward to taking you to the park again. I love you very much.

Family and Friends

Whether related by blood or marriage, the reaction of family and friends to the new mother's depression can critically affect her recovery.

Sometimes a depressed mother feels too inhibited to tell her partner about uncomfortable feelings, fearing disapproval. This mom may open up to you first, if given an opportunity. But even if she is talking openly with her partner, having the right kinds of support from those including her parents, in-laws, grandparents, siblings, and friends, will provide her with the optimal environment for recovery.

When we become mothers, even if we aren't depressed, we often crave the company and approval of our own mothers. If the woman's own mother is deceased, or if their relationship is strained, it will be extra important to have another woman who can help fill that void. Because depressed mothers are, in general, even more vulnerable than non-depressed mothers, they will need substantial reassurance from those around them, especially from adult females.

New moms in general are sensitive to criticism. Moms with postpartum mood disorders are typically even more sensitive. Compliment her frequently on her mothering and avoid negative comments, especially those related to her parenting.

Things to Keep in Mind

- *You will not be able to cure her.*
  You may feel frustrated that postpartum illnesses cannot be cured in the same way as other conditions. The course of this illness, even with medication, is different from that of an ear infection, for example. Where most common conditions get steadily better until they disappear, postpartum illnesses fluctuate during recovery.

  Typically the woman advances two steps forward and feels better, and then drops one step back and "dips." She may feel despondent and hopeless when these dips occur, since depression robs her of a perspective that she is getting well. She may voice that she is back to square one and that she is not getting better.

  It is important that you remind her that the dip is only temporary, she is getting better, and her moods will get back on track. A dip is not a regression — it is simply part of the process. Remind her that as long as she is going in the right direction overall, that is what is most important.

- *Encourage, do not insist.*
  Women suffering from postpartum depression often feel incapable of finding the words to communicate their feelings. While it is positive to encourage her to share her thoughts, it is unhelpful to demand it. Let her know you are willing to listen without judging her.

  Trust that she will open up when she is ready and feels what she has to say will be treated seriously and respectfully. Even just being there in total silence together can be a great support. Your presence alone is tremendously helpful, even if she cannot or chooses not to speak.

- ***Stay in the here and now.***
  With her moods fluctuating, the recovering woman cannot trust that the good times will last. She never knows when her brain chemistry will shift and her moods will drop. She may be reluctant to share the good times with you for fear that you'll think she no longer needs your support.

  Eventually the good times will last and the dips will go away, but this process can take several weeks or even months. Reassure her that you understand she will be riding some waves in mood for a while, and that your support won't be suddenly yanked away before she's ready.

- ***Don't let looks fool you.***
  Postpartum depression is a hidden illness. These women often appear normal to the outside world. They can look "put together," complete with makeup, jewelry, and even a smile, and be deeply depressed at the same time.

  Sometimes the more depressed a mom feels, the more she overcompensates for it on the outside. For instance, if she feels ashamed, she may try to act perky in order to hide her true feelings. It is important to ask the mother how she is doing and never assume based on how she appears. So if you hear another family member say, "But she doesn't look depressed," you can teach them that looks can be quite deceiving when it comes to postpartum illness.

What to Say, What Not to Say

Say:

- *I'm here for you.*
- *I'm sorry you are suffering. That must feel awful.*
- *You're doing a great job.* Be specific whenever you can.
- *You're a great mom.* Give specific examples, like "I love how you smile at the baby."
- *You're a great... (sister, daughter, aunt).* Be specific.
- *You will get well.*
- *Would you like me to do... (insert task)*
- *I went through this, too.* If you truly did — remember, this is not "Baby Blues" and will not go away in a few days.

Do Not Say:

- *Just buck up and tough it out.*
  Not getting adequate treatment puts women at risk of chronic illness and relapse.
- *I don't get what the big deal is.*
  Depression makes everything feel like a big deal. She's overwhelmed.
- *You have so much to be happy about.*
  She knows that already. She feels guilty that she is still depressed despite those things.
- *You just need more sleep.*
  Sleep is important, but is usually not all she needs to be well.
- *You just need a break from your baby.*
  Breaks are crucial, but usually not all that is needed.

- *I went through this too.*
  This is not "Baby Blues." Don't minimize her experience by saying you've "been there" unless you really have suffered with this illness.
- *Women have been having babies for centuries.*
  And a certain percentage has been getting depressed for centuries!

What you can do to help

- Make dinner.
- Watch the baby (or her other children) so she can take a break.
- Do the laundry.
- Do the dishes.
- Make lunch for her.
- Sit and listen.
- Clean the house.
- Take a walk together.
- Go shopping or do errands for her.
- Write thank you notes for her.
- If her partner is not home, be on duty at night so she can sleep.

SIX

Health Practitioners

The fact that you are reading this book clearly indicates that you are a caring and concerned professional. Your guidance during this critical time will significantly impact the mental and physical well-being of women with perinatal mood disorders. It is important not to underreact or overreact to these women's symptoms. Just treat them as matter-of-factly as you would any other common perinatal experience, for example, gestational diabetes.

This chapter contains answers to the questions that we have been most frequently asked throughout the years regarding signs, symptoms, and treatment. Because a distressed woman's contact with a professional office includes the receptionist and nursing staff, it is imperative that the entire staff be know-ledgeable about the information in this book. We have created sections for primary care providers (family practitioners, internists, osteopaths, chiropractors), pediatricians, OB/GYNs and midwives, psychiatrists, birth doulas, postpartum doulas and visiting nurses, lactation consultants, childbirth educators, new parent group leaders, and adjunct professionals.

Please remember that warning signs of distress are not always obvious for a variety of reasons. Shame, guilt, or fear of judgment may cause the woman to hide her feelings. She may present more "socially acceptable" complaints such as fatigue, headache, marital problems, or a fussy baby. Just because a woman is smiling or well groomed, don't assume she is not suffering silently. Postpartum depression is a hidden illness. Although there are risk factors to help predict postpartum depression, there is no particular "type" of person who becomes afflicted.

We appreciate that you may be apprehensive about asking questions that could open a Pandora's box. She might feel accused of being a bad mom, and become defensive. But once she hears your matter-of-fact tone, and understands no shame is attached to postpartum illness, she will be able to accept the information. In the long run, you will be saving time and providing quality care.

Culture and Language

Although the prevalence of perinatal mood disorders appears to be generally the same throughout the world, reactions to these disorders vary among cultures. Where shame is a great personal threat, for example, women may be more reluctant to discuss their symptoms and will require considerable reassurance.

Those assisting women with these disorders should take into account that nonverbal communication varies among cultures as well. For instance, a nod could signify either understanding or acquiescence to authority. It is also important to make clear what your role is in order to avoid unrealistic expectations.

Sociocultural factors and literacy levels should not be overlooked when taking a history or completing an assessment. The perception of stress, types of stressors, as well as coping styles, differ across cultures. These will affect the woman's response to recommendations on which treatment methods to use or to avoid.

The level of simplicity or sophistication you use should be attuned to that of the patient, but do not assume that an educated woman will automatically understand her condition better than a woman with less education. For instance, avoid raising questions of self-diagnosis, such as, "Do you think you have postpartum depression?" even when a patient is highly educated. She may have a preconceived idea of what that term means. Instead, ask specific questions about her mood and behavior, which will elicit this information. These questions are outlined later in this chapter.

What to Say, What Not to Say

Say:

- *These feelings are quite common.*
- *This is treatable.*
- *You will get well.*
- *Here is some information that will help you.*

Do Not Say:

- *Join a new mom's group.*
  If a mother is clinically depressed or anxious, this may be a damaging suggestion, depending largely on the leader of the group. A depressed mother is already feeling different and inadequate compared to other new mothers. Attending a "normal" new mothers' group may intensify her alienation.

  If you know that the leader of the group is sensitive (such as those reading this book) and discusses mood problems, this mom will be fine. Ideally, she should join a group specifically designed for mothers with postpartum depression and anxiety. Many of our clients belong to both types of groups: one to discuss the normal new mom stuff and the other to openly express more difficult feelings.

- *Take a vacation with your husband.*
  Although a change of scenery may be nice, the depressed mother takes her brain chemistry with her! Her anxiety and depression level may actually increase due to the financial investment, leaving her baby, and guilt that the trip did not "cure" her.

- *Exercise.*
  These mothers are feeling overwhelmed. Some have barely enough energy to wash a bottle, let alone go to the gym. Suggesting exercise to the chronically sleep-deprived mother can actually backfire and cause insomnia. Endorphins only work temporarily. Exercise will not cure her depression. When she's able to leave her house and take a short walk, she can be encouraged to do so. But, until then, this is just another setup for failure.

- *Do something nice for yourself.*
  This is always a good thing, but again, it will not be enough to regulate the depressed mother's neurotransmitters. This suggestion should be used only as part of a much larger treatment plan, not presented as a quick fix.

- *Sleep when the baby sleeps.*
  Even a non-depressed mother may have difficulty sleeping when the baby naps during the day. Especially for those mothers with high levels of anxiety, this will be an impossibility. What is most important is that she sleeps at night when her baby sleeps.

Screening

We recommend whenever possible using standardized screening surveys, such as the Postpartum Depression Screening Scale or the Edinburgh Postnatal Depression Scale. For your immediate use, we have outlined informal screening tools. We use the term "perinatal psychotherapist" to indicate a psychotherapist who specializes in the field of perinatal mood disorders.

Prenatal Screening

Several prenatal screening inventories have been developed. They are listed in the resource section. If time is too limited to use screening questionnaires, the questions in the **Pre-pregnancy and Pregnancy Risk Assessment** should be asked. At the bare minimum, the questions associated with highest measure of risk must be asked, noted with a ★. These are the questions relating to personal/family history of mental illness, previous postpartum mood disorder, and severe premenstrual mood changes.

Given prenatally, the Edinburgh Postnatal Depression Scale has been found to effectively identify women at risk for postpartum depression.

PRE-PREGNANCY AND PREGNANCY
RISK ASSESSMENT

Warning Signs

- Missed appointments
- Excessive worrying (about her own health or health of fetus)
- Looking unusually tired
- Crying
- Requires support person to accompany her to appointments
- Significant weight gain or loss
- Physical complaints with no apparent cause
- Flashbacks, fear, or nightmares regarding previous trauma
- Her concern that she won't be a good mother

Questions to Ask   ★ *These indicate high risk.*

Note: Even if your clients/patients have experienced these disorders, they may not be aware of this fact if they were never formally diagnosed. You may need to ask about their experience with the symptoms of the disorders as opposed to using diagnostic terms in order to adequately assess.

★ *Have you ever had depression, panic, extreme anxiety, OCD, bipolar disorder, psychosis, or an eating disorder?* Women with a personal history of mood disorders need to be educated about their high risk for a perinatal mood disorder. They should be referred to a perinatal psychotherapist to help them develop a plan of action to minimize their risk. Those women with a history of bipolar disorder or psychosis should also be referred to a psychiatrist for medication evaluation and observation during pregnancy and postpartum.

★ *Are you taking any medications (prescription or nonprescription) or herbs on a regular basis?*
Women who are self-treating for insomnia, anxiety, sadness or other symptoms that may indicate a mood disorder, should be evaluated by a perinatal psychotherapist.

★ *Have you had a previous postpartum mood disorder?*
Women answering yes to this question are at extremely high risk for another perinatal mood disorder. They should be referred to a perinatal psychotherapist in order to develop a plan of action to prevent or at least minimize another occurrence.

★ *Have you ever taken any psychotropic medications?*
If yes, educate them about their risk of developing a perinatal mood disorder. Observe them carefully during pregnancy and postpartum.

★ *Have you ever had severe premenstrual mood changes (PMS or PMDD)?*
Women whose moods are affected by hormone changes are clearly at high risk during pregnancy and postpartum since there are dramatic hormonal shifts. Educate them about their risk, and observe them carefully during pregnancy and postpartum.

★ *Do you have any family history of mental illness?*
If yes, educate them about their risk, and observe them during pregnancy and postpartum.

• *Do you have any personal or family history of substance abuse?*
• *Do you smoke?*

- *If pregnant, how have you been feeling physically and emotionally?*
- *Do you feel you have adequate emotional and physical support?*
- *Have you had a birth-related trauma (or other traumatic incident such as rape or sexual abuse)?*
- *Are you experiencing any major life stressors (for example, moving, job change, deaths, financial problems)?*
- *Have there been any health problems for you or the fetus?*
- *Do you have a personal or family history of thyroid disorder?*

Postpartum Screening

Two postpartum depression screening inventories are available (see Resources). Either one can easily be completed in a waiting room.

The Edinburgh Postnatal Depression Screening Scale (EPDS) was developed in 1987 in Britain, by Dr. John Cox, et al. It is a 10 question self-report test. It has been translated into many languages and is used all over the world. It can be found on many Internet sites.

More recently, Dr. Cheryl Beck has developed the Postpartum Depression Screening Scale (PDSS). It has been found to accurately screen for both postpartum depression and anxiety. The PDSS can be administered in either a short or long format. The total score can be broken down into seven symptom content scales when using the long format. An elevated score in a particular symptom area indicates a greater amount of distress than average. The symptom scales are: Sleeping/Eating Disturbances, Anxiety/Insecurity, Emotional Lability, Mental Confusion, Loss of Self, Guilt/Shame, and Suicidal Thoughts.

In comparing the PDSS with the EPDS, Beck found that the PDSS has higher combinations of specificity and sensitivity than the EPDS in screening for major postpartum depression. Additionally, the PDSS was more likely to identify women with symptoms of sleep disturbance, mental confusion, and anxiety. If you have assessed that a woman has a postpartum mood disorder, here are some basic "do's and don'ts."

POSTPARTUM RISK ASSESSMENT

With your postpartum patients who were not screened prenatally, ask the first six questions from the **Pre-pregnancy and Pregnancy Risk Assessment** (the questions marked with ★), as well as the **Postpartum Risk Assessment.**

Warning Signs in the Mother
- Missed appointments
- Excessive worrying (often about the mother's own health or health of baby)
- Looking unusually tired
- Requires support person to accompany to appointments
- Significant weight gain or loss
- Physical complaints with no apparent cause
- Poor milk production (could indicate thyroid dysfunction)
- Evading questions about her own well-being
- Crying
- Not willing to hold baby or unusual discomfort handling or responding to baby
- Not willing to allow others to care for baby
- Excessive concern about baby despite reassurance (for example, eating sufficiently, development, weight gain)

- Rigidity or obsessiveness (for example, regarding the baby's feeding or sleeping schedules)
- Excessive concern about appearance of self or baby
- Expressing that baby doesn't like her or that she's not a good mother
- Expressing lack of partner support

Warning Signs in the Baby

- Excessive weight gain or loss
- Delayed cognitive or language development
- Decreased responsiveness to mother
- Breastfeeding problems

Questions to Ask

- *How are you doing?*
  Have good eye contact with her while you ask this question.

- *How are you feeling about being a mom?*
  Women who feel like they're doing a bad job or who generally don't like the job, may be depressed.

- *Do you have any particular concerns?*

- *How are you sleeping (quality and quantity)?*
  Five hours minimum of uninterrupted sleep per night is required for a complete sleep cycle, necessary to restore brain chemistry.

- *Can you sleep at night when everyone else is asleep?*
  Insomnia is a symptom of every mood disorder.

- *How is the baby sleeping?*

- *Who gets up at night with the baby?*

- *Have you had any unusual or scary thoughts?*
  If yes, refer woman to a perinatal psychotherapist for evaluation. Some thoughts may be normal, however others may indicate OCD or psychosis.

- *Are you receiving adequate physical and emotional help?*
  A good support system of family and friends can make a significant difference.

- *Is your partner sharing the responsibilities of household and parenting?*
  Remind her that these jobs do not just belong to her, even if she is the primary caretaker.

- *Do you generally feel like yourself?*
  Women with postpartum mood disorders often report not feeling like their usual selves, or having a different personality.

- *How is your appetite?*
  A significant change in appetite is a warning sign.

- *What and how often are you eating and drinking?*
  See section on eating in Chapter 3.

- *If breastfeeding, how is it going?*
  Poor milk production may indicate a thyroid dysfunction or be a result of anxiety.

- *If using formula, when and how quickly did you wean?*
  Abrupt weaning can precipitate a mood disorder.

- *When was your last period?*
  First menses after delivery can be a precipitating factor.

- *Are you taking any medications or herbs on a regular basis?*
  Women who are self-treating for insomnia, anxiety, sadness or other symptoms which may indicate a mood disorder, should be evaluated by a perinatal psychotherapist.

- *Are you feeling moodier than normal (tearful, irritable, or worried)?*
  This is common in mood disorders. Refer to Chapter 2 for a more complete list of symptoms.

- *Have there been any health problems for you or the baby?*
  These factors increase the risk for mood disorders.

- *How are you feeling toward your baby?*
  Ambivalence and anger are two examples of feelings that may indicate postpartum depression.

Primary Care Providers

As a primary care provider, you may have a longstanding relationship with your patient. You have a good sense of her mental and physical health history. This puts you in an advantageous position to evaluate her pre-pregnancy risk, and provide appropriate direction. Your office may provide a safe haven should a pregnancy or postpartum mood problem arise. Please have information from the Resource section available, as well as local referrals.

A woman taking psychotropic medications who is pregnant or planning a pregnancy should be encouraged to consult a psychiatrist specializing in perinatal mood disorders in order to determine whether to continue her medications. Recommendations will differ based on each woman's history and symptomatology. Women on medication for a bipolar disorder or psychosis should definitely be referred to a psychiatrist to develop a medication plan. These women need careful monitoring throughout pregnancy and postpartum.

Use the **Pre-pregnancy and Pregnancy Risk Assessment** on ALL women who are pregnant or planning a pregnancy. Even if she is feeling fine early in the pregnancy, she may not later in pregnancy or postpartum. She should be screened periodically throughout the pregnancy.

With your postpartum patients who were not screened prenatally, ask the first six questions from the **Pre-pregnancy and Pregnancy Risk Assessment** (the questions marked with ★), as well as the **Postpartum Risk Assessment.**

Use the **Postpartum Risk Assessment** on ALL women during their first year postpartum.

Pediatricians

The well-being of your patient is largely dependent on the well-being of the primary caregiver, usually the mother. It is well documented that the mental health of the mother has a tremendous impact on the emotional and physical development of the child. While the focus of the pediatric visit is primarily the baby, the health of the mother is a crucial component that must not be overlooked.

In addition to the obvious milestones, the mother-baby relationship must be assessed. She will need your reassurance if she wishes to nurse while taking an antidepressant. Have local referrals and information in the Resources section available.

If you have the opportunity to screen the woman before her baby is born, ask at least the first six questions from the **Pre-pregnancy and Pregnancy Risk Assessment** (the questions marked with ★).

Use the **Postpartum Risk Assessment** at every well baby visit throughout the first year postpartum for ALL your patients' mothers.

OB/GYNs and Midwives

Your office has been a source of comfort and advice throughout the pregnancy. This intimate relationship makes it likely that a woman with postpartum distress will come to you for help if she feels depressed or anxious. However, many women will not be forthcoming with negative feelings or concerns unless specifically asked. Have local referrals and information in the Resources section available. Please follow up on a regular basis.

A woman taking psychotropic medication who is pregnant or planning a pregnancy should be encouraged to consult a psychiatrist specializing in perinatal mood disorders to determine whether to continue or change her medication. Recommendations will differ based on each woman's history and symptomatology. Women on medication for a bipolar disorder or psychosis should definitely be referred to a psychiatrist to develop a medication plan. These women need careful monitoring throughout pregnancy and postpartum.

Use the **Pre-pregnancy and Pregnancy Risk Assessment** on ALL women who are pregnant or planning a pregnancy. Even if she is feeling fine early in the pregnancy, she may not later in pregnancy or postpartum. She should be screened periodically throughout the pregnancy.

With your postpartum patients who were not screened prenatally, ask the first six questions from the **Pre-pregnancy and Pregnancy Risk Assessment** (the questions marked with ★) as well as the Postpartum Risk Assessment.

Use the **Postpartum Risk Assessment** on ALL women during their first year postpartum.

Psychiatrists

Since you are the professionals who work most closely with psychotropic medications, many perinatal women will be referred to you for assessment and treatment of mood disorders. You play an integral role in this treatment team.

Research findings and recommendations about medications in pregnancy and lactation are constantly changing. There have been some important findings recently in the area of medication management of perinatal mood disorders, which will be discussed later in this text. If you are only providing medication management, make sure you give your patients the name of a psychotherapist trained in perinatal mood disorders.

Use the **Pre-pregnancy and Pregnancy Risk Assessment** on ALL your patients who are pregnant or planning a pregnancy.

Use the **Postpartum Risk Assessment** on ALL women during their first year postpartum.

Birth Doulas

Studies show that the use of a doula contributes to the reduction of postpartum depression. As a birth doula, you are in a unique position to screen prenatally for risk and to watch for early warning signs of emotional problems. If, for instance, when administering the **Pre-pregnancy and Pregnancy Risk Assessment**, you discover the woman has suffered a previous traumatic delivery or childhood sexual abuse, she may experience flashbacks during the upcoming birth. Have local referrals and information in the Resources section available.

A woman taking psychotropic medication who is pregnant or planning a pregnancy should be encouraged to consult a psychiatrist (specializing in perinatal mood disorders) in order to determine whether to continue her medication. Recommendations will differ based on each woman's history and symptomatology. Women on medication for a bipolar disorder or psychosis should definitely be referred to a psychiatrist to develop a medication plan. These women need careful monitoring throughout pregnancy and postpartum.

If you are interviewed before employment, you can ask her if she has any particular concerns about birthing or postpartum. She then may share some information which could give you clues about her mental health. Let the woman know that one of your strengths is sensitivity to the various emotions which can occur during birth and postpartum.

Use the **Pre-pregnancy and Pregnancy Risk Assessment** on ALL women who employ your services. If you continue to see these women postpartum, use the **Postpartum Risk Assessment.** Keep in mind that this information can be gathered quite informally, simply through chatting. Be familiar with the questions and the pertinent information you need in order to screen.

Postpartum Doulas and Visiting Nurses

You have the opportunity to observe the home and social environments of the mother, which can give crucial information about her well-being and that of the family unit. For instance, if you notice a lack of partner support or signs of marital conflict, she is at greater risk for a postpartum mood disorder. If her house is unusually neat and clean, you will want to find out who is doing the housework. If she is, for example, obsessively cleaning or awake in the middle of the night vacuuming, this is not normal. Have local referrals and information in the Resources section available.

If you are just meeting women postpartum, you have not had the opportunity to screen them prenatally. Ask the first six questions from the **Pre-pregnancy and Pregnancy Risk Assessment** (the questions marked with ★), as well as the **Postpartum Risk Assessment.**

As long as you are familiar with the questions and understand what information you're trying to gather, this screening can be accomplished very informally through chatting.

Women should be assessed throughout the first year. If your last visit to her is before one year postpartum, make sure she has referral information in case she needs it later.

Women already on medication, or those who you assess need a medical evaluation, should be referred to a psychiatrist specializing in perinatal mood disorders.

Lactation Consultants

The role of a lactation consultant may superficially appear to be one-dimensional and relate only to the mechanics of breastfeeding. However, as we know, you are also providing tremendous emotional support. You may be the first professional to see the mother and baby during the initial postpartum weeks.

Your intimate relationship with the mother at this vulnerable time allows you to observe and listen for potential emotional problems. Postpartum moms listen carefully to what you advise and are quite trusting of you. It is so important that you help each woman decide what is right for her.

If her physical or emotional health is declining, it is obviously not good for the baby. You have a great deal of influence as to whether new mothers give themselves permission to take care of themselves (for instance, five hours of uninterrupted sleep at night). Sometimes this will mean partial or complete weaning.

Difficulty breastfeeding is associated with postpartum depression and anxiety, and also thyroid dysfunction. When a woman is weaning her baby, make sure she weans her own body very slowly even though her baby can wean "cold turkey."

Abrupt weaning can precipitate a mood disorder, especially when a woman is predisposed. If she is already suffering, abrupt weaning can greatly exacerbate her symptoms. Especially if a woman is depressed and not feeling good about herself, there can be a great amount of guilt if at any point she cannot or should not continue breastfeeding. What you say or do not say at that time can make a big difference regarding how she feels about herself as a mother.

Many professionals are unaware of the current research regarding nursing and psychotropic medications. It is important that you are informed so you can advocate for women who want to nurse while taking medication. Have local referrals and information in the Resources section available, including a psychiatrist who has experience prescribing medication during lactation.

Your assessment of ALL women not previously screened should consist of the first six questions from the **Pre-pregnancy Risk Assessment** (the questions marked with ★), plus the **Postpartum Risk Assessment.** As long as you are familiar with the questions and understand what information you're trying to gather, much of the screening can be completed quite informally through chatting.

Childbirth Educators

So often we hear the lament, "Why didn't anyone warn us in our birthing classes about mood problems during and after pregnancy?" Even though your primary focus is on labor and delivery, you have a responsibility and opportunity to educate couples about perinatal mood disorders. This might be a difficult topic to discuss since no woman wants to think it could happen to her.

If you know a professional who is an expert in this field, you can invite her or him to speak to your class. If not, bring the subject up in a matter-of-fact manner, the same way you would any other common pregnancy or postpartum experience.

The rate of depression in pregnancy is 10 percent. Therefore, we can assume some of the women in your classes are already suffering and are at risk for a postpartum mood disorder. Your participants will not bring up this topic, so you need to. There is no danger in giving information, and there is great danger in omitting it. You have a captive audience with both members of the couple. The partner might be soaking up this information even if the mother-to-be is not. It is often the spouse who later recognizes the symptoms and encourages his wife to seek help.

Hand out some information from the Resources section and the name and number of a professional trained in perinatal mood disorders. At the class reunion ask about participants' feelings about the challenges as well as the joys of parenthood. Be sure to call participants who did not attend the reunion. They may not be doing well and could be trying to avoid an uncomfortable situation.

New Parent Group Leaders

If there are ten women in your group, remember that, statistically, at least one of them will have postpartum depression. Rarely will this woman be brave enough to disclose her feelings, since she will most likely be experiencing guilt and shame. She will be aching for someone to open the door to this discussion and give her permission to express how she is really feeling. If spouses and fathers are present, ask them how they are doing.

Encourage discussion about the normal feelings accompanying adjustment to parenting and the relationship to oneself, partner, baby, friends, and family. You can easily work in some facts about moods and behaviors that fall outside the realm of normal adjustment.

For each new group, make sure this topic gets explored in a nonjudgmental manner. If you prefer, you can invite a professional with expertise in this area to lead a discussion. In any case, use the information in the Resources section and the names and numbers of local professionals trained in the area of postpartum disorders.

Adjunct Professionals

There are many other wonderful professionals who touch the lives of pregnant and postpartum women. For example, physical therapists and instructors in prenatal and postpartum exercise should mention the possibility of mood disorders, since you are encountering suffering women all the time. Above all, making the information in the Resources section available will support the pregnant and postpartum women with whom you work.

SEVEN

Treatment

At the top of the list are the most important treatment methods: information and education. She needs to know her illness has a name, and is treatable. Depending on the severity and cause(s) of her symptoms, sometimes this is all a woman needs in order to recover. This information may come from professionals, nonprofessionals, or both.

Alternative Therapies

Studies are currently being conducted regarding the treatment of depression in pregnancy and postpartum which do not involve medication.

For instance, the therapeutic effect of massage on depression in pregnancy and postpartum is beginning to emerge in the data. Morning bright light therapy is already being used both in pregnancy and postpartum either as an alternative or in conjunction with medication. Compelling evidence about the effectiveness of the Omega-3 essential fatty acid DHA (docosahexaenoic acid) in both the prevention and treatment of postpartum depression is also apparent. Taken while nursing, the baby's neurological development may also be enhanced.

Some therapies are not yet found in the literature as proven treatments; however, many of our clients have used them, including acupuncture, homeopathic remedies, chiropractic, Yoga, hypnotherapy and types of spiritual and energy healing. We advocate using the therapy or combination of therapies (including medication) which is the most effective for each individual. In other words, use whatever is safe and works!

Women seeking treatment often try to alleviate symptoms on their own before seeking the advice of a professional. This self-treatment may include potentially risky substances, such as alcohol or untested herbal or drug remedies. Little research has been done on the safety of herbs such as St. John's wort during pregnancy or nursing.

Herbs can be wonderful but they can also be dangerous. They are powerful medicines, often produced with little or no regulation or safety monitoring. Some herbal remedies and illegal drugs have been associated with serious harm to both mother and child, including birth defects, infant death, and liver toxicity. On the other hand, quite a bit of research has been conducted regarding the use of certain prescription medications during pregnancy and lactation that effectively combat perinatal mood disorders.

The most immediate goal of treatment is to alleviate suffering as quickly as possible. While it is generally prudent to start medication at a low dosage, it should be increased as rapidly as possible to whatever the therapeutic dosage is for that woman. Undertreating can lead to chronic symptomatology and increase the risk of relapse.

What follows here are guidelines only. All treatment must be individualized. For medication management we recommend the woman see a psychiatrist with expertise in treating perinatal mood disorders.

Since brand names may vary by country, we are including both brand and generic names of medications.

Pregnancy

I have spent the last 10 years of my career worrying about the impact of medications. I've been wrong. I should have been worrying more about the impact of illness.

ZACHARY STOWE, MD
ASSISTANT PROFESSOR, DEPARTMENT OF PSYCHIATRY, EMORY UNIVERSITY

Current thinking regarding the use of medications in pregnancy has evolved over the past few years. Researchers who have spent years investigating the potential effects of medication on the fetus have shifted their focus to the harmful effects on the fetus when maternal mental illness goes untreated. These experts agree that maternal depression and anxiety must be evaluated and treated to maximize a positive outcome for the baby.

Pregnancy causes alterations in metabolism and blood volume; therefore, higher doses of medications may be required to reach therapeutic levels.

Antidepressants

Studies of selective serotonin reuptake inhibitors (SSRIs) or tricyclics (TCAs) used in pregnancy have revealed no increased risk of physical malformations, neonatal complications, miscarriage, or impairments in neurobehavioral development. At seven years of age exposed children tested normally on IQ and development tests. These data include first trimester exposure.

Based on current research, the preferred choices during pregnancy are Prozac and Sarafem (fluoxetine), Zoloft (sertraline), Paxil (paroxetine) and Celexa (citalopram). The top researchers maintain that there is no reason to change from one medication to another; go with what works and gets the quickest results.

Electroconvulsive Therapy (ECT)

ECT is considered an acceptable treatment for severe depression or psychosis in pregnancy. It may also be useful in treating bipolar disorder during pregnancy. ECT is not an appropriate treatment for prenatal anxiety, panic, or obsessive-compulsive disorder (OCD).

Antipsychotics

Conventional high-potency antipsychotics, such as Haldol (haloperidol), are recommended over low-potency or atypical agents throughout pregnancy.

Mood Stabilizers

Recent research shows that the risk of Ebstein's (cardiac) anomaly with lithium use in the first trimester is under 1 percent. In one study no significant neurobehavioral or developmental problems were noted. A fetal cardiac ultrasound between weeks 18 and 20 is recommended for those with first trimester exposure. Lithium maintenance throughout pregnancy should be considered for women with severe bipolar disorders, since the risk of relapse is high. Reintroducing lithium after discontinuation in the first trimester does not protect well against relapse. Other mood stabilizers, such as Tegretol (carbamazepine) and Depakote (valproic acid), increase the rate of neural tube defects and are not recommended during pregnancy.

Antianxiety Medications

The literature regarding antianxiety exposure in utero is limited and confusing. First trimester use has been associated with cleft palate. However, women with anxiety or panic disorder should be treated. SSRIs, while not specifically antianxiety medications, are effective in treating these disorders. Ativan (lorazepam) is used for short-term relief of symptoms. The lowest effective dose for the shortest period of time is recommended.

Sleep Aids

If sleep is impaired due to depression or anxiety, medication may be necessary. TCAs such as Pamelor (nortriptyline) or Elavil (amitriptyline) may be useful at bedtime. Deseryl (trazadone) also has a sedative effect. Ambien (zolpedem) has a faster rate of onset and is considered acceptable in pregnancy.

Postpartum

Thyroid

At least 10 percent of postpartum women will develop postpartum thyroiditis. In the early stages of thyroiditis, women may experience anxiety or depression. Sometimes this condition is temporary, and will resolve without treatment in about six months. But for others it can lead to chronic thyroiditis and hypothyroidism (Hashimoto's thyroiditis).

Since thyroid disorders can cause depression and anxiety, thyroid dysfunction must be ruled out. The suggested time for testing is between two and three months postpartum. The following tests are recommended for all women with postpartum mood complaints: free T4, TSH, anti-TPO, and anti-thyroglobulin. It is important to check for the anti-thyroid antibodies (anti-TPO and anti-thyroglobulin) since there have been many cases where the T4 and TSH levels were within normal ranges but the anti-thyroid antibody titers were elevated. We recommend that the woman be evaluated by an endocrinologist if she has thyroid abnormalities.

Hormone Therapy

Hormone therapy for postpartum depression is still being evaluated for efficacy. Research with estrogen holds promise for treatment of postpartum depression and postpartum psychosis. Taking estrogen, like any medicine, has certain risks and needs to be evaluated on a case-by-case basis.

Women sensitive to hormonal shifts, including those with postpartum depression and anxiety who choose oral contraceptives (birth control pills), need to be monitored closely for mood changes. Women may experience fewer mood problems on a monophasic birth control pill as compared to a triphasic birth control pill. The monophasic pill delivers the same ratio of estrogen and progesterone unlike the triphasic, where the ratio changes weekly.

Women with a history of increased moodiness on oral contraceptives should consider alternate methods of contraception. Synthetic progesterone (progestin) has been associated with a worsening of symptoms. Depo-Provera (medroxyprogesterone acetate), a long-acting progesterone injection, is not a good option since it cannot be discontinued should it aggravate mood problems. Hormone therapy is not currently recommended as sole treatment for postpartum psychiatric disorders.

Medications

A woman who is not nursing has a vast arsenal of medications available to her. If this woman, or a blood relative, has had a positive experience with any particular medication, that would be the first choice.

Few studies have been done on the efficacy of particular medications in the treatment of postpartum depression/anxiety.

One study published in 2001 did find Effexor (venlafaxine) to be effective in the treatment of postpartum depression. Wellbutrin (bupropion) for postpartum women with depression but without anxiety seems to be energizing and also reduces the likelihood of sexual side effects.

There is not one medication that, in general, is better than the others for treating postpartum depression. In our experience all the SSRIs work well. Each woman has her own individual chemistry which will work better with certain medications than with others. It is prudent to start with a low dose and follow up regularly, increasing the dosage until an adequate therapeutic response is achieved. She should report feeling back to "herself." Under-treating can lead to chronic illness and increased risk of relapse.

Medications and Nursing

There are no good data to support any particular antidepressant (with lithium as an exception) being safer than another for women suffering from depression who wish to breastfeed.

LEE S. COHEN, MD
DIRECTOR, PERINATAL AND REPRODUCTIVE PSYCHIATRY PROGRAM
MASSACHUSETTS GENERAL HOSPITAL
ASSOCIATE PROFESSOR OF PSYCHIATRY, HARVARD MEDICAL SCHOOL

Antidepressants

Antidepressants of choice (based on the available research) for lactating mothers are Zoloft (sertraline), Paxil (paroxetine), TCAs (tricyclic antidepressants), Prozac and Sarafem (fluoxetine), and Celexa (citalopram). The first choice for every woman should be a medication that has worked for her in the past or one that has been used successfully with a blood relative.

The benefits of nursing far outweigh the theoretical risks of medications. The amounts of metabolites found in the infant's serum are so small they are almost impossible to detect. Behaviorally and developmentally these infants and children are normal.

Mood Stabilizers

Tegretol (carbamazepine) and Depakote (valproic acid) are approved by the American Academy of Pediatrics (AAP) for breastfeeding mothers. Lithium is not recommended.

Antipsychotics

High-potency antipsychotics, such as Haldol (haloperidol), are used for nursing moms.

Sleep Aids

Ambien (zolpedem), Restoril (temazepam), Deseryl (trazadone), Pamelor (nortriptyline), or Elavil (amitriptyline) are frequently prescribed for nursing moms.

Antianxiety Medications

Low doses of short acting medications such as Xanax (alprazolam) or Ativan (lorazepam) can be used on an occasional as-needed basis for anxiety, panic, and sleep.

Electroconvulsive Therapy (ECT)

ECT is considered an acceptable treatment for severe depression or psychosis postpartum, including for nursing mothers. It may also be useful in treating bipolar disorder postpartum. ECT is not an appropriate treatment for postpartum anxiety, panic, or OCD.

Medical Protocols

The chart below suggests treatments based upon the woman's history. Treatments should be followed in sequence, with Treatment 1 tried first, followed by Treatment 2 if necessary.

Although the treatment protocols that follow refer only to depression and psychosis, they are also effective in the treatment of OCD, anxiety and panic.

SSRIs are usually the first line medications in the treatment of OCD, anxiety and panic. For OCD, Luvox (fluvoxamine) and Anafranil (clomipramine) are second choices. Although Anafranil tends to have more side effects, it seems to be acceptable during pregnancy and lactation. Luvox has not been as well studied for use in pregnancy or lactation. It may be helpful to use low dose anti-anxiety medications on a short-term basis for anxiety and panic.

Pre-Pregnancy		
History	**Treatment 1**	**Treatment 2**
One episode of major depression if on medication + asymptomatic for 6–12 months	Taper off medication + psychotherapy (monitor closely for relapse)	Resume medication + continue psychotherapy
Severe recurrent prior episodes	Continue medication + psychotherapy	
Mild major depression	Psychotherapy	Psychotherapy + medication
Severe major depression (first episode)	Medication + psychotherapy	
Bipolar disorder	Continue or switch to lithium + monitor closely by psychiatrist + psychotherapy	Switch to high potency antipsychotic if lithium-resistant or intolerant + continue psychotherapy

Pregnancy (including first trimester)		
History	**Treatment 1**	**Treatment 2**
One episode mild major depression, currently in remission	Trial slow tapering medication + psychotherapy	Resume medication + psychotherapy
One episode severe major depression, currently in remission	Maintenance on medication + psychotherapy	
Mild major depression, first or recurrent	Psychotherapy	Medication + psychotherapy*
Severe major depression, first episode	Medication + psychotherapy	ECT + psychotherapy
Recurrence or relapse of depression if off medication if mild major depression	Psychotherapy	Resume medication + psychotherapy
Severe major depression, currently symptomatic	Resume medication + psychotherapy	ECT + psychotherapy
Psychosis in any trimester *Note: do not rely on psychosocial interventions alone; requires hospitalization.*	Antipsychotic + psychotherapy Add mood stabilizer or antidepressant if needed once stable Or ECT + psychotherapy	

If this is not successful, further treatment of ECT + psychotherapy should be considered.

Postpartum		
History	**Treatment 1**	**Treatment 2**
Mild major depression	Psychotherapy	Psychotherapy + medication
Severe major depression	Psychotherapy + medication	Consider ECT
Postpartum psychosis *Note: hospitalization required. Do not rely on psychosocial interventions alone.*	Antipsychotic + psychotherapy Add mood stabilizer or antidepressant if needed once stable Or ECT + psychotherapy	

Prevention of Postpartum Depression in Women with History of Depression, Anxiety, Other Mood Disorder, or Prior PPD		
History	**Treatment 1**	**Treatment 2**
First pregnancy	Meet with psychotherapist when risk identified (pre-pregnancy or pregnancy) + psychoeducation for woman and partner	Intervention (refer to pregnancy treatment protocol) if symptomatic
Prior postpartum depression	Psychoeducation for woman and partner as early as possible + start antidepressant 2–4 weeks before delivery + psychotherapy Or start anti-depressant immediately after delivery + psychotherapy	
Prior postpartum psychosis	Start lithium upon delivery + psychotherapy	

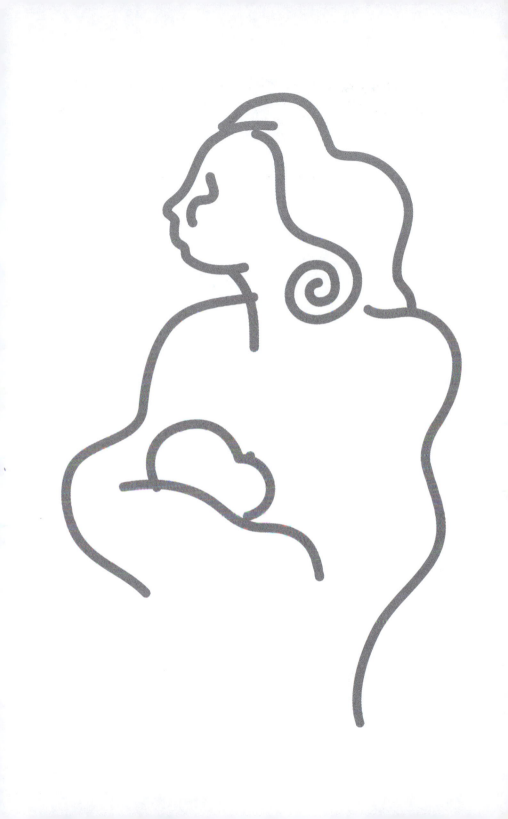

EIGHT

Resources

Organizations

Depression After Delivery
(800) 944-4PPD
www.depressionafterdelivery.com
Answering machine. Will send packet on PPD with some resources.

The Marcé Society
PO Box 30853
London, England W12OXG
www.marcesociety.com
International organization dedicated to scientific research in the field.
Annual conference.

National Hopeline Network
609 E. Main St., #112
Purcellville, VA 20132
(800) SUICIDE (784-2433)

North American Society for Psychosocial OB/GYN
409 12th Street, S.W.
Washington, DC 20024-2188
(202) 863-1628
www.naspog.org
Annual conference.

Postpartum Health Alliance (California's State organization)
20052 Jessee Ct.
Castro Valley, CA 94552
(510) 889-6017
www.postpartumhealthalliance.org
Semi-annual training on diagnosis and treatment of perinatal mood disorders.

Postpartum Support International
(805) 967-7636
www.postpartum.net
Telephone support and international directory of members.
Annual conference.

Websites

American Family Physician, Postpartum Major Depression:
Detection and Treatment
www.aafp.org/afp/990415ap/2247.html

Baby Center, Postpartum Depression
www.babycenter.com/refcap/227.html

British Columbia Reproductive Mental Health Program's
Reading Room
www.bcrmh.com/disorders/postpartum.htm

Canadian Pacific Postpartum Support Society
www.postpartum.org

Center for Postpartum Health
www.postpartumhealth.com

Childbirth and Postpartum Professional Association
www.childbirthprofessional.com

Depression After Delivery
www.depressionafterdelivery.com

Depression Central
www.psycom.net/depression.central.post-partum.html

Doulas and Postpartum Caregivers
www.childbirth.org/doula123.html

Doulas of North America
www.dona.org

Duke University: Your Emotional Well-being: Understanding the Blues
www.duke.edu/%7Ebkc/html/webdoc7.htm

The Marcé Society
www.marcesociety.com

Massachusetts General Hospital, Center for Women's Mental Health
www.womensmentalhealth.org/

Medlineplus Health Information
www.nlm.nih.gov/medlineplus/postpartumdepression.html

National Association of Postpartum Care Services
www.napcs.org

New Zealand, Bounty Services
www.bounty.co.nz

North American Society for Psychosocial OB/GYN
www.naspog.org

Postpartum Assistance for Mothers
www.postpartumassistance.com

Postpartum Depression and Caring for Your Baby
www.kidshealth.org/parent/pregnancy_newborn/home/ppd_baby.html

Postpartum Depression Online Support Group
www.ppdsupportpage.com

Postpartum Education for Parents
www.sbpep.org

Postpartum Health Alliance
www.postpartumhealthalliance.org

Postpartum Resource Center of New York, Inc.
www.postpartumny.org

Postpartum Support International
www.postpartum.net

Pregnancy and Depression Medical Articles
www.pregnancyanddepression.com

Ruth Rhoden Craven Foundation, Inc. for Depression Awareness
www.ppdsupport.org

South Africa
www.pndsa.co.za

UCLA Mood Disorders Research Program
www.npi.ucla.edu/uclamdrp/pregnantpostpart.htm

Books

Dunnewold, Ann. *Evaluation and Treatment of Postpartum Emotional Disorders.* Sarasota, Florida: Professional Resource Press, 1997.

Dunnewold, Ann, and Diane Sanford. *Postpartum Survival Guide.* Oakland, California: New Harbinger Press, 1994.

Fran, Renee. *What Happened to Mommy?* (Can be ordered for $7.95 payable to Renee, from R.D. Eastman, P.O. Box 290663, Brooklyn, N.Y. 11229.)

Hanson, Rick, Hanson, Jan, and Ricki Pollycove. *Mother Nurture: A Mother's Guide to Health in Body, Mind, and Intimate Relationships.* New York: Penguin Books, 2002.

Honikman, Jane. *Step by Step, A Guide to Organizing a Postpartum Parent Support Network in Your Community.* 927 N. Kellogg Ave., Santa Barbara, CA 93111.

Honikman, Jane. *I'm Listening: A Guide to Supporting Postpartum Families.* 927 N. Kellogg Ave., Santa Barbara, CA 93111

Kendall-Tackett, Kathleen, and Glenda Kantor. *Postpartum Depression: A Comprehensive Approach for Nurses.* Newbury Park, California: Sage Publications, 1993.

Klaus, Marshall, Kennell, John, and Phyllis Klaus. *The Doula Book: How a Trained Labor Companion Can Help You Have a Shorter, Easier, and Healthier Birth.* Cambridge, Massachusetts: Perseus Publishing, 2002.

Kleiman, Karen. *The Postpartum Husband.* Philadelphia: Xlibris, 2000.

Kleiman, Karen, and Valerie Raskin. *This Isn't What I Expected: Overcoming Postpartum Depression.* New York: Bantam Books, 1994.

Miller, Laura, ed. *Postpartum Mood Disorders.* Washington, D.C.: American Psychiatric Press, 1999.

Misri, Shaila. *Shouldn't I Be Happy? Emotional Problems of Pregnant and Postpartum Women.* New York: Free Press, 1995.

Nicholson, et. al, *Parenting Well When You're Depressed; A Complete Resource For Maintaining a Healthy Family.* Oakland: New Harbinger Publications, Inc., 2001.

Placksin, Sally. *Mothering The New Mother.* New York: Newmarket Press, 1994.

Raskin, Valerie. *When Words Are Not Enough: The Women's Prescription for Depression and Anxiety.* New York: Broadway Books, 1997.

Roan, Sharon. *Postpartum Depression: Every Woman's Guide to Diagnosis, Treatment, and Prevention.* Hollbrook, Massachusetts: Adams Media Corporation, 1997.

Robin, Peggy. *Bottlefeeding Without Guilt: A Reassuring Guide for Loving Parents.* Roseville, California: Prima Publishing, 1996.

Sebastian, Linda. *Overcoming Postpartum Depression and Anxiety.* Omaha: Addicus Books, 1998.

Sichel, Deborah, and Jeanne Driscoll. *Women's Moods.* New York: William Morrow and Co., 1999.

Steiner, Meir, and Kim Yonkers. *Depression in Women: Mood Disorders Associated with Reproductive Cyclicity.* Pfizer, Inc., 1998.

Treatment of Depression in Women 2001, Postgraduate Medicine: A Special Report. The Expert Consensus Guideline Series. White Plains, NY: Expert Knowledge Systems. (Can be ordered from the publisher at 21 Bloomingdale Rd., White Plains, NY, 10605 for $12.95.)

Tronick, E.Z., and Tiffany Field. *Maternal Depression and Infant Disturbance.* San Francisco: Jossey-Bass, 1987.

Tronick, E. Z., Cohn, J., Shea, E. *The Transfer of Affect Between Mothers and Iinfants.* In T. B. Brazelton and M. W. Yogman (eds.) Affective Development in Infancy. Norwood, NJ: Ablex. 1986; 11-25.

Journal Articles

Prenatal Screening

Beck, C. A checklist to identify women at risk for developing postpartum depression. *J Obstet Gynecol Neonatal Nurs.* Jan-Feb 1998; 27(1):39-46.

Posner, N., et al. Screening for postpartum depression; an antepartum questionnaire. *J Reprod Med.* 1997; 42:207-215.

Postpartum Screening

Cox, J.L., et al. Detection of postnatal depression: development of the 10-item Edinburgh Postnatal Depression Scale. *British Journal of Psychiatry.* 1987; 150:782-786.

Beck, Cheryl Tatano, and Robert Gable. Postpartum Depression Screening Scale (PDSS). Available through Western Psychological Services (800) 648-8857.

Postpartum Depression

Cohen, L.S., et al. Venlafaxine in the treatment of postpartum depression. *J Clin Psychiatry.* 2001; 62(8):592-596.

Hendrick, V., et al. Postpartum and nonpostpartum depression: differences in presentation and response to pharmacologic treatment. *Depression and Anxiety.* 2000; 11:66-72.

Hibbeln, J.R. Seafood consumption, the DHA content of mother's milk and prevalence rates of postpartum depression: a cross-national, ecological analysis. *J Affective Disorders.* 2001.

Nonacs, R., and Cohen, L.S. Postpartum mood disorders: diagnosis and treatment guidelines. *J Clin Psychiatry.* 1998; 59 (suppl 2):34-40.

Stowe, Z.N. and Nemeroff, C.B. Women at risk for postpartum-onset major depression. *Am J Obstet Gynecol* 1995 Aug; 173(2):639-644.

Depression in Pregnancy

Hendrick, V., Altshuler, L. Management of major depression during pregnancy. *Am J Psychiatry.* 2002 Oct; 159(10):166-173.

Oren, D.A., et al. An open trial of morning light therapy for treatment of antepartum depression. *Am J Psychiatry.* 2002 Apr; 159(4):666-669.

Medications During Pregnancy

Altshuler, L., et al. Pharmacologic management of psychiatric illness during pregnancy: dilemmas and guidelines. *Am J Psychiatry.* 1996 May; 153:592-606.

American Academy of Pediatrics. Use of Psychoactive Medication During Pregnancy and Possible Effects on the Fetus and Newborn. *Pediatrics.* 2000 Apr; 105(4): 880-887.

Barki, J., Kravitz, H., Berki, T. Psychotropic medications in pregnancy. *Psychiatric Annals.* 1998 Sep; 28:486-497.

Baugh, C., and Stowe, Z. Treatment issues during pregnancy and lactation. *CNS Spectrums,* 1999 Oct; 4(10); 34-39.

Cohen, L. Pharmacologic treatment of depression in women: PMS, pregnancy, and the postpartum period. *Depression and Anxiety.* 1998; 8(suppl 1):18-26.

Cunningham, M., and Zayas, L.H. Reducing depression in pregnancy: designing multimodal interventions. *Soc Work.* 2002 Apr; 47(2):114-23.

Kulin, N., et al. Pregnancy outcome following maternal use of the new selective serotonin reuptake inhibitors. *JAMA.* 1998; 279(8):609-610.

Nonacs, R., Cohen, L.S. Depression during pregnancy: diagnosis and treatment options. *J Clin Psychiatry.* 2002; 63 (suppl 7):24-30.

Nulman, I., et al. Neurodevelopment of children exposed in utero to antidepressant drugs. *NEJM.* 1997; 336 (4):258-262.

Pinelli, J.M., Symington, A.J., Cunningham, K.A., Paes, B.A. Case report and review of the perinatal implications of maternal lithium use. *Am J Obstet Gynecol.* 2002 Jul;187(1):245-249.

Wisner, K.L. et al. Pharmacologic treatment of depression during pregnancy. *JAMA.* 1999; 282:1264-1269.

Medications and Lactation

Birnbaum, C. S., et al. Serum concentrations of antidepressants and benzodiazepines in nursing infants: a case series. *Pediatrics.* 1999; 104:11.

Burt, V.K., et al. The use of psychotropic medications during breastfeeding. *Am J Psychiatry*. 2001; 158:1001-1009.

Chaudron, L. When and how to use mood stabilizers during breastfeeding. *Primary Care Update OB/GYNs*. 2000; 7(3).

Chaudron, L., and Jefferson, W. Mood stabilizers during breastfeeding: a review. *J Clin Psychiatry*. 2000; 61:79-90.

Llewellyn, A., and Stowe, Z. Psychotropic medications in lactation. *J Clin Psychiatry*. 1998; 59(suppl 2):41-52.

Stowe, Z., et al. Paroxetine in human breast milk and nursing infants. *Am J Psychiatry*. 2000; 157:185-189.

Suri, R. A., et al. Managing psychiatric medications in the breastfeeding woman. *Medscape Women's Health*. 1998; 3(1).

Wisner K.L., et al. Antidepressant treatment during breastfeeding. *Am J Psychiatry*. 1996; 153(9):1132-1137.

Psychotherapy

Appleby, L., et al. A controlled study of fluoxetine and cognitive-behavioural counseling in the treatment of postnatal depression. *BMJ*. 1997; 314:932-936.

Beck, C.T., A meta-analysis of predictors of postpartum depression. *Nurs Res*. 1996; 45:297-303.

O'Hara, M.W., Stuart, S., Gorman, L.D., Wenzel, A. Efficacy of interpersonal psychotherapy for postpartum depression. *Arch Gen Psychiatry*. 2000; 57(11): 1039-1045.

Spinelli, M.G., Interpersonal psychotherapy for depressed antepartum women: a pilot study. *Am J Psychiatry*. 1997; 154:1028-1030.

Effects of Maternal Depression on Children

Beck, C. T. Maternal depression and child behaviour problems: a meta-analysis. *J of Advanced Nursing.* 1999; 29, 623-629.

Field, Tiffany. Maternal depression effects on infants and early interventions. *Preventive Medicine.* 1998; 27:200-203.

Field, Tiffany. Emotional care of the at-risk infant: early interventions for infants of depressed mothers. *Pediatrics.* 1998 Nov; 102(5) (suppl):1305-1310.

Gelfland, D., Teti, D. The effects of maternal depression on children. *Clinical Psycholog Review.* 1990; 10:329-353.

Glover, V., O'Connor, T.G. Effects of antenatal stress and anxiety: Implications for development and psychiatry. *Br J Psychiatry.* 2002 May; 180:389-391.

Goodman, S. H., Adamson, A. B., Riniti, J., Cole, S. Mothers' expressed attitudes: associations with maternal depression and children's self-esteem and psychopathology. *J A Acad Child Adolesc Psychiatry.* 1994; 33:1265-1274.

Miller, L., et al. Self-esteem and depression: ten-year follow-up of mothers and offspring. *J of Affective Disorders.* 1999; 52:4-49.

Newport, D.J., Hostetter, A., Arnold, A., Stowe, Z.N. The treatment of postpartum depression: minimizing infant exposures. *J Clin Psychiatry.* 2002; 63 (suppl 7):31-44.

Orr, Suzanne T., James, Sherman A., Prince, Cheryl Blackmore. Maternal prenatal depressive symptoms and spontaneous preterm births among African-American women in Baltimore, Maryland. *Am J Epidemiol.* 2002; 156:797-802.

Appendix:
Medical Terms and
Healthcare Professionals

Medical Terms	
Bipolar Disorder	Also known as manic depression, this is a chemical imbalance in the brain characterized by moodswings from manic (see "mania") to depressed. Many researchers believe there is a strong genetic component to this illness.
Cognitive Behavioral Therapy (CBT)	With CBT, the therapist takes an active role in the therapy process and provides a clear structure and focus to treatment. Behavior therapy helps the client weaken the connections between situations and the negative habitual reactions to them. Cognitive therapy teaches the client how certain thought patterns or beliefs create symptoms such as depression, anxiety or anger. The therapist works with the client to help develop new positive ways of thinking and acting.
Cortisol	Called the "stress hormone," cortisol is a hormone released by the adrenal glands during anxious or agitated states.
Delusion	This is a false belief. One may fear being pursued or think she is someone other than herself. Often there is religious content to the thoughts.

Depression	A common disorder characterized by sad mood, irritability, sleep and appetite disturbances, loss of pleasure, fatigue, and hopelessness. Depression can be caused by a variety of factors, including biochemical, emotional, and psychological.
Etiology	The cause or origin of a disease or illness.
Hallucination	Something one sees or hears that others do not. Hallucinations often have religious overtones, for example, hearing the voice of God or Satan.
Insomnia	Inability to sleep.
Interpersonal Psychotherapy (IPT)	IPT is a brief and highly structured psychotherapy that addresses interpersonal issues. IPT helps the client solve problems, for instance, disputes, feeling isolated, adjusting to new roles, or grief following a loss. The therapist works from a collaborative framework.
Mania	A symptom of bipolar disorder (see above) characterized by exaggerated excitement, hyperactivity, and racing, scattered thoughts. A person in a manic state feels an emotional "high" and often does not use good judgment. Speech may be rapid and she may feel little need for sleep or food. Thinking is usually confused and she may act in sexually, socially, and physically unhealthy ways, for instance, inappropriate sexual behavior or shopping sprees.
Mood Instability	When moods fluctuate and change rapidly. Mood may swing from happy to sad, for instance.
Neurotransmitter	Chemical released by nerve cells that carries information from one cell to another. This type of chemical transmits messages in the brain. Some neurotransmitters are serotonin, norepinephrine, and dopamine.

Obsessive-Compulsive Disorder (OCD)	Occurs in about 1 in 4 people. OCD is associated with a chemical imbalance in the brain. This condition worsens in times of stress. Obsessions are thoughts which occur intrusively and repetitively (for instance, thoughts of the baby being harmed). Compulsions are repetitive actions which often take the form of cleaning, checking (for instance, the locks on the door or the baby's breathing), or counting (for instance, the number of diapers in the bag). A person may have only obsessions, or a combination of the two.
Panic Disorder	During a panic attack, the person may feel symptoms including intense fear, rapid breathing, sweating, nausea, dizziness, and numbness or tingling. Sufferers often fear having the next panic attack and may develop behaviors to avoid situations thought to put them at risk.
Perinatal Mood Disorder	A mood disorder (for instance, depression or anxiety) beginning during pregnancy or during the first year postpartum.
Phobia	A persistent, irrational fear of a specific object, activity, or situation. This fear usually leads either to avoidance of the feared object or situation, or to enduring it with dread. Common phobias include fear of heights, flying in airplanes, fear of small places, and spiders.
Postpartum	After a mother gives birth.
Posttraumatic Stress Disorder (PTSD)	PTSD can occur following life-threatening or injury producing events such as sexual abuse or assault, or traumatic childbirth. People who suffer from PTSD often experience nightmares and flashbacks, have difficulty sleeping, and feel detached. Symptoms can be severe and significantly impair daily life.

Premenstrual Dysphoric Disorder (PMDD)	About 3 to 8% of women experience severe mood changes around their periods that create a significant impact on relationships and lifestyle. There are now specific diagnostic criteria that define this disorder.
Premenstrual Syndrome (PMS)	A combination of symptoms that appears the week before a menstrual period, and resolves within a week after the onset of the period. Common symptoms include: bloating, cramping, irritability, fatigue, anger, and depression. About 75% of women experience some degree of PMS.
Prenatal	During pregnancy.
Psychoanalysis	A form of psychotherapy that focuses on unconscious factors affecting current relationships and patterns of behavior, traces the factors to their origins, shows how they have changed over time, and helps the client cope with adult life. The client talks and the therapist is primarily a listener. Usually therapy takes place four or five times a week, and can continue for years.
Psychosis	An extreme and potentially dangerous (suicide, infanticide) mental disturbance which includes losing touch with reality. The psychotic person displays irrational behavior, has hallucinations and delusions. Hospitalization and medication are required.
Psychotropic Medication	Medication that affects thought processes or feeling states by acting on brain chemistry. Antidepressants and antianxiety medications are included in this category.

Healthcare Professionals

Note: Licensure varies from state to state. Also, information about perinatal mood disorders is not a routine part of most training programs. See section in Chapter 3 on finding a knowledgeable therapist.

Certified Midwife (CM)	A CM is an individual educated in the discipline of midwifery, who is certified by the American College of Nurse-Midwives. The CM provides primary healthcare to women including: prenatal care, labor and delivery care, care after birth, gynecological exams, newborn care, assistance with family planning, preconception care, menopausal management and counseling in health maintenance.
Certified Nurse-Midwife (CNM)	A CNM is a licensed healthcare practitioner educated in nursing and midwifery. She provides primary healthcare to women of childbearing age including: prenatal care, labor and delivery care, care after birth, gynecological exams, newborn care, assistance with family planning, pre-pregnancy care, menopausal management, and counseling in health maintenance. CNMs attend over 9% of the births in the United States. Many CNMs are able to prescribe medication.
Clinical Psychologist	Mental health professionals who have earned a doctoral degree in Psychology (either a Ph.D., Psy.D, or Ed.D). They have received extensive clinical training in research, assessment, and the application of different psychological therapies. Clinical psychologists are concerned with the study, diagnosis, treatment, and prevention of mental and emotional disorders. They are not able to prescribe medication.

Doula	The doula's role is to provide physical and emotional support to women and their partners during labor and birth. Some doulas are also trained in postpartum care. The doula is not a labor coach. Her main role is to provide emotional reassurance and comfort. Doulas do not perform clinical tasks such as vaginal exams or fetal heart rate monitoring. Doulas are not trained to diagnose medical or psychological conditions or give medical advice.
Endocrinologist	A physician (MD) who specializes in treating problems related to hormones. Endocrinologists frequently treat thyroid problems.
Lactation Consultant	Trained, often certified, specialist who provides support and education about the process of breastfeeding. A Lactation Consultant can provide help regarding nursing, pumping, bottlefeeding, and weaning.
Licensed Clinical Professional Counselor (LCPC)	An LCPC is a masters level mental health professional. LCPCs are not able to prescribe medications.
Marriage and Family Therapist (MFT)	A masters level license in California, MFTs are similar to LCSWs and LCPCs. They are trained in individual, couple, and family therapy. MFTs are not able to prescribe medication.
Midwives, other *(See Certified Nurse-Midwife & Certified Midwife)*	Some women practice midwifery without a license. Be sure to ask about training and licensure.

Psychiatrist	These mental health professionals have earned the MD (Medical Doctor) degree. Advanced training focuses on psychiatric diagnosis, psychopharmacology (medication management of mental health issues) and psychotherapy. These physicians are the experts in prescribing psychotropic medications.
Psychiatric Nurse (APRN)	Registered Nurses who seek additional education and obtain a masters or doctoral degree can become Advanced Practice Registered Nurses in a specialty (APRNs). They provide the full range of psychiatric care services to individuals, families, groups, and communities, and in most states they have the authority to prescribe medications. APRNs are qualified to practice independently.
Psychiatric Social Worker	These mental health professionals have earned the MSW (Masters in Social Work) degree and are trained to be sensitive to the impact of environmental factors on mental disorders. LCSW designates Licensed Clinical Social Worker. These professionals cannot prescribe medication.
Psychotherapist	A person who practices psychotherapy: either a clinical psychologist, psychiatrist, professional counselor, social worker, or other mental health professional. Unless this person is also an MD (medical doctor), he/she cannot prescribe medication.

INDEX

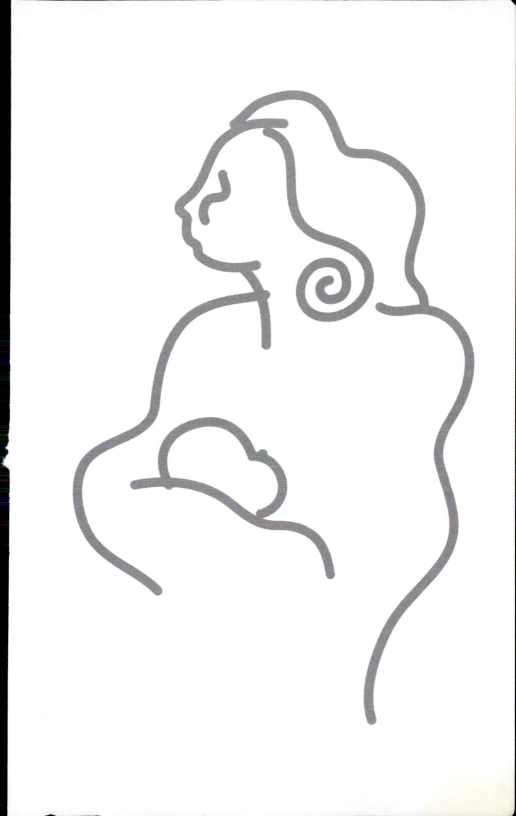

QUICK ORDER FORM

Beyond the Blues
A Guide to Understanding and Treating
Prenatal & Postpartum Depression

Order by Internet:
www.beyondtheblues.com
Credit cards accepted over the Internet

Order by mail:
Send your check or money order to:
Moodswings Press, 1050 Windsor St., San Jose, CA 95129-2837

Name: _____

Address: _____

City: _____ State: _____ Zip: _____

Telephone: _____ Email: _____

Quantity: _____ @ $14.95 per book $ _____

Sales Tax:

California residents please add 7.25% $ _____

Shipping:

Add $3.00 shipping for 1 book, $ _____

then $1.00 for each additional book $ _____

Total Enclosed: $ _____

PLEASE ALLOW 7-10 BUSINESS DAYS FOR DELIVERY

CONTACT US FOR BULK DISCOUNT RATES
books@beyondtheblues.com • Fax (408) 246-0217